T0332024

Dramatherapy with Children, Young People and Schools

Dramatherapy with Children, Young People, and Schools is the first book to specifically evaluate the unique value of dramatherapy in the educational environment. A variety of highly experienced dramatherapists, educational psychologists and childhood experts discuss the benefits to the children and young people, and also in relation to the involvement of teachers, the multi-disciplinary team and families, This professional book offers a panoramic view to explain how through dramatherapy children and young people develop their communication skills, sociability and their actual desire to learn.

Detailed case studies demonstrate individual successes in youngsters experiencing a range of emotional difficulties and psychological needs. These studies include: conquering a fear of maths; violent behaviour transformed into educational achievement; safe expression of feelings for a sexually abused child; and where children are diagnosed with mental health disorders such as ADHD and ODD, where the benefits of dramatherapy with children and families are carefully described and evaluated, suggesting that this therapeutic discipline can achieve positive outcomes.

The practical advice and inspirational results included here promote a future direction of integration and collaboration of school staff, multi-disciplinary teams and families. Education and equality are high on the agenda, and the function of dramatherapy is not just as a treatment, but as an economically viable and valuable preventive therapy.

Lauraine Leigh is a dramatherapist and teacher who has worked over 18 years with a range of children in the NHS and in mainstream and special schools and units, with behavioural difficulties, special needs and mental health diagnoses, promoting close communication with and support of parents and teachers around the child.

Irvine Gersch is Professor of Educational and Child Psychology at the University of East London (UEL). He is a chartered educational psychologist and chartered scientist. He is a Fellow of the British Psychological

Society, The Royal Society of Arts and the Higher Education Academy. He is the Programme Director for the Professional Doctorate in Applied Educational and Child Psychology at UEL and a Director of Global Mediation.

Ann Dix is a freelance dramatherapist and supervisor. Prior to this she was manager of a multi-agency support team in Leeds, working with schools, children and families. Ann was a drama teacher before qualifying as a dramatherapist in 1993.

Deborah Haythorne is the co-founder and co-director of Roundabout, the largest dramatherapy charity in the UK. Deborah qualified as a drama-therapist in 1985 and completed her research on dramatherapy with children with autistic spectrum disorder in 1996.

"I recommend this book to every dramatherapist, to every teacher, and to every health care administrator, because within its pages lies a vision of the future of education that we cannot afford to postpone. The many authors of chapters span the academic, clinical, educational, and research fields. This is an important book!" – *David Read Johnson, Ph.D., RDT-BCT, Director, Institutes for the Arts in Psychotherapy New York; Co-Director, Post Traumatic Stress Center New Haven, Connecticut; Associate Clinical Professor Department of Psychiatry, Yale University School of Medicine.*

This is "a timely, comprehensive and accessible book; essential reading for dramatherapists working in schools and also for teachers, teaching assistants, learning mentors and others engaged in education. The complexities and difficulties in the lives of many children and young people are sensitively described and the creative practices of those writing will offer inspiration to all." – *Pat Broadhead, Professor of Playful Learning, Leeds Metropolitan University.*

This is "an essential book for anyone working in education and especially government who are changing policies and funding. The book gives a clear exposition of the educational practice of dramatherapy and the underlying theories. Educational psychologists will understand the vital contribution that dramatherapy makes for children with learning, behavioural and emotional needs. The book is clearly and concisely written without jargon, that makes it accessible for teachers and therapists alike. It is also a very good read!" – *Professor Sue Jennings, International Dramatherapist and author.*

This book is "thoroughly rewarding. It clearly describes how troubled pupils can be effectively helped, so that they are less stressed, have more fun and achieve better educational outcomes. The dramatherapy practice is a very welcome source of inspiration." – *Dr. Alida Gersie, author of books about Storymaking and Change and freelance education consultant.*

"This book provides an insightful exploration of the role of dramatherapy with children, young people and schools. The content highlights the creativity and commitment involved in approaching this work with clear links to the evidence supporting dramatherapy as an important intervention for young people experiencing a range of difficulties. Case studies and clinical examples provide the reader with an authentic sense of the work, lending itself to clinical application for those working in the field." – *Vicky Baldwin, Education & Practice Consultant, Institute of Mental Health.*

This is "a campaigning book aimed at many different audiences, waving the flag for dramatherapy at a time when resources are scarce but new possibilities are arising in how schools are run.

The basic argument is that emotional learning is as important as academic learning. The book conveys how dramatherapy combines psychoanalytic understanding with physical and imaginative play in a way that engages directly with how the child experiences things. The case studies demonstrate how arts therapies like dramatherapy can help a troubled child or young person to manage their unruly or suppressed emotions in a way that allows them to achieve their full learning potential". – *David Kennard, Head of Psychology and Psychotherapy at The Retreat, York; Director of the Tuke Centre for Psychotherapy and Counselling; group analyst; author.*

"Dramatherapists have been working in schools for many years supporting vulnerable children and young people. I am delighted that we now have a book that discusses this work in such an interesting and informative way. (This book will be). . . a great resource for trainee therapists, other professionals and parents." – *Marian Lindkvist, Former Director and Founder of The Sesame Institute UK and International.*

"The ideal of creativity is entering the mainstream of language, becoming a goal in education. It discusses the magic of who we are and our connection and co-creation with the universe." – *Marcia Karp International and UK Psychodramatist and author.*

Dramatherapy with Children, Young People and Schools

Enabling Creativity, Sociability, Communication and Learning

Edited by Lauraine Leigh, Irvine Gersch, Ann Dix, and Deborah Haythorne

Routledge
Taylor & Francis Group
LONDON AND NEW YORK

First published 2012 by Routledge
27 Church Road, Hove, East Sussex, BN3 2FA

Simultaneously published in the USA and Canada
by Routledge
711 Third Avenue, New York NY 10017

Routledge is an imprint of the Taylor & Francis Group, an Informa business

© 2012 Selection and Editorial matter Lauraine Leigh, Irvine Gersch, Ann Dix, and Deb Haythorne; Individual chapters, The Contributors

All rights reserved. No part of this book may be reprinted or reproduced or utilised in any form or by any electronic, mechanical, or other means, now known or hereafter invented, including photocopying and recording, or in any information storage or retrieval system, without permission in writing from the publishers.

Trademark notice: Product or corporate names may be trademarks or registered trademarks, and are used only for identification and explanation without intent to infringe.

British Library Cataloguing in Publication Data
A catalogue record for this book is available from the British Library

Library of Congress Cataloging-in-Publication Data
Dramatherapy with children, young people, and schools : enabling creativity, sociability, communication and learning / edited by Lauraine Leigh . . . [et al.].
p. cm.
Includes bibliographical references and index.
1. Drama–Therapeutic use. 2. Child psychotherapy. 3. Adolescent psychotherapy. I. Leigh, Lauraine.
RJ505.P89D735 2012
618.92'89142–dc23
2011027898

ISBN: 978-0-415-67076-0 (hbk)
ISBN: 978-0-415-67077-7 (pbk)

Typeset in Times by Garfield Morgan, Swansea, West Glamorgan
Paperback cover design by Lisa Dynan; cover image: Sydney Klugman

MIX
Paper from responsible sources
FSC
www.fsc.org
FSC® C004839

Printed and bound in Great Britain by
TJ International Ltd, Padstow, Cornwall

Dedication

This book is dedicated to Oscar, Alfie, Francie, Natty, Pheobe and Isla, Jacob, Aaron, Ben, Jonathan and Bertie and all children and young people growing now. . .

And in loving memory of Ray and Eileen Sharp.

. . . and so everyone according to his cue.

A Midsummer Night's Dream, III. i

By the stars too are men guided

Sura XVI – The Bee, The Koran

Contents

Contributors

Madeline Andersen-Warren is a dramatherapist, supervisor and trainer. She was Chair of The British Association of Dramatherapists from 2004 to 2010. Her publications include 'Therapeutic Theatre' in *Dramatherapy Clinical Studies* (edited by Steve Mitchell; Jessica Kingsley 1995), *Practical Approaches to Dramatherapy* (with Roger Grainger; Jessica Kingsley 2000) and 'Theatre Model of Dramatherapy Supervision' in *Supervision of Dramatherapy* (with Anna Seymour, edited by Ditty Dokter and Phil Jones; Routledge 2009). She is completing doctoral research in dramatherapy.

Tamar Brown works as a clinical psychologist and family therapist in the adolescent unit of a psychatric hospital in southern France. She co-founded and works as a trainer using dramatherapy for the association Cerma-Psyche. She trained initially as an actress, then as a drama-therapist and in psychoanalytical studies at the Tavistock Clinic. Her work experience since 1991 has primarily been in child psychiatry. Since 2010, she has run a dramatherapy module within the arts therapy training course at IRFAT in Avignon, France. With representatives from several European countries, she plans a European Dramatherapy Association.

Talya Bruck trained as a speech and drama teacher in her native South Africa before embarking on her dramatherapy training in the UK, where she also trained as a clinical supervisor. She has worked extensively in primary and secondary schools as well as Pupil Referral Units. Currently Talya works as part of a Child and Adolescent Mental Health Services team in schools as well as running a private practice.

Mandy Carr is a dramatherapist, arts therapies supervisor and teacher who has set up dramatherapy in primary, secondary and special educational settings. Currently the convenor of BADth's Equality and Diversity Sub-Committee, she has recently completed research into cross-cultural awareness within dramatherapy. Mandy's interests include performance poetry and world music. She co-wrote a chapter in *Supervision in Dramatherapy* (edited by D. Dokter and P. Jones, Routledge 2008).

Alyson Coleman is a dramatherapist, lecturer and supervisor. She currently works within the NHS and as a lecturer at Central School of Speech and Drama on the MA Drama and Movement Therapy (Sesame) training. Her doctoral research looks at the area of dramatherapy and childhood bereavement.

Geoffrey Court taught in primary schools and adult education for 12 years. His special interests as a class teacher were music, and the life of the class as a group. The Playground Project transformed his view of children and their capabilities. Long experience as a tutor in a psychiatric social club was another rich source of learning. In 1985 he established an organisation that offers reflective space to people working in the community, The Circle Works, whose name reflects to this day the deep influence of the Magic Shop.

Susan Crockford is the North London coordinator for Roundabout, which includes work as a dramatherapist and supervisor, and developing evaluation methods. She is also employed as a dramatherapist in the NHS and has worked with a variety of client groups including children and young people in mainstream education and special schools.

Ann Dix trained as a drama teacher and taught in a Northampton upper school and a large children's home before becoming a dramatherapist. She has also studied family therapy and play therapy. Ann is manager of a multi-agency team in Leeds and works with children and families. She is a registered clinical supervisor.

Ditty Dokter is head and professional lead arts psychotherapies at the Hertfordshire Partnership NHS Foundation Trust and course leader MA Dramatherapy at Anglia Ruskin University. She has many years of clinical and training experience in a variety of settings. Her research interest is in intercultural and evidence-based practice. She recently coordinated the systematic review of practice-based evidence for the British Association of Dramatherapists. Her most recent publications are P. Jones and D. Dokter (eds) (2008) *Supervision in Dramatherapy*, 'Embodiment in Dramatherapy' in P. Jones (ed.) (2010) *Drama as Therapy* vol. 2 and several chapters in D. Dokter, P. Holloway and H. Seebohm (eds) (2011) *Dramatherapy and Destructiveness*, all published by Routledge.

Dolmen Domikles has worked as a dramatherapist in adult mental health and child and adolescent mental health, both in London and the South. He presently works as a primary mental health worker (CAMHS) for Sussex Partnership Foundation NHS Trust. He has a Level 1 Practitioner qualification from the Institute of Developmental Transformations in New York, and is a founder member of the DvTUK steering group. He heads DCT training workshops in East Sussex.

Roya Dooman has worked for over 20 years as a dramatherapist for Social Services, schools, hospices and charities in the UK and abroad. Her interest in bereavement led her to co-create a project for children affected by HIV and AIDs in South London. She currently works in inner-city primary schools, supervises therapists and lectures on the MSc Therapeutic Counselling Course at Greenwich University.

Professor Irvine Gersch is Professor of Educational and Child Psychology at the University of East London (UEL). He is a chartered educational psychologist and chartered scientist. He has worked as a teacher, principal educational psychologist, university lecturer and programme director. He has acted as advisor to the Department of Education, the National Audit Office, and consultant to a number of local authorities. He is a Fellow of the British Psychological Society, The Royal Society of Arts and the Higher Education Academy, and Programme Director for the Professional Doctorate in Applied Educational and Child Psychology at UEL and a Director of Global Mediation.

His research and publications have been in the area of special needs, listening to children, school systems, mediation and arts therapies, and the use of philosophy, mindfulness and spirituality with children. Currently, he is leading a project to develop spiritual listening tools and techniques for use by psychologists and other practitioners.

Emma Godfrey is a lecturer in psychology at King's College London and a state-registered dramatherapist. She is currently programme leader for the Intercalated BSc in Psychology and teaches a range of health professionals. Her research interests include mental health in children and young people and the interface between mental and physical health.

Jennifer Greene is an educational psychologist working for a local authority in London. Jennifer has worked with children diagnosed with an autism spectrum disorder (ASD) and their families since 2004, and is currently developing a specialism in ASD.

Rex Haigh consultant psychiatrist, Berkshire Healthcare NHS Foundation Trust; Clinical Advisor, National Personality Disorder Programme and Senior Fellow, Institute of Mental Health, University of Nottingham is founder and project lead of the 'Community of Communities' quality network at the royal college of Psychiatrists. Involved with third-sector organisations including the Association of Therapeutic Communities, Borderline UK, Personality Plus, Community Housing and Therapy, the Society for Psychotherapy Research and the British and Irish Group for the Study of Personality Disorder, he has written and published numerous articles about therapeutic communities and personality disorder and is co-editor of both the Jessica Kingsley *Community, Culture and Change* book series and the *International Journal of Therapeutic Communities*.

Deborah Haythorne is an HPC registered dramatherapist and a British Association of Dramatherapists registered dramatherapy supervisor. She is the co-founder and co-director of Roundabout, the largest dramatherapy charity in the UK. Deborah qualified as a dramatherapist in 1985 and completed her research on dramatherapy with children with autistic spectrum disorder in 1996. She has taught on the MA Dramatherapy courses at the Central School of Speech and Drama and at Roehampton University. She has pioneered the use of 'PSYCHLOPS Kids' in Roundabout's school projects.

Jeff Higley has worked in the arts as a performer, sound artist and sculptor for over 30 years, devising and directing large-scale public events and performances for many organisations, including the Barbican Centre, the South Bank Centre, WWF and Festival of Sacred Earth Drama. He has completed many Public and Community Art commissions working as a wood sculptor and has continued to perform in the Colourscape touring inflatable installation as part of the group Hyperyak. A deep interest in ecology and the relation of humans to other species led to his becoming Chair and later online Editor for the Landscape and Arts Network – www.landartnet.org

Dimpi Hirani trained at the Sesame Institute in 2003. Since then she has worked as a dramatherapist in a number of special needs schools. Currently she works for Respond with children and young people with learning disabilities who have experienced sexual abuse and domestic violence. She also provides training to professionals and parents around sexual abuse issues. Her special interest lies in working with young people with autism. She appeared in the Channel 4 documentary 'Young, Autistic and Stagestruck' in April/May 2010.

Clive Holmwood studied drama and educational theatre at the University of Leeds. After working for some time as a freelance drama practitioner he trained as a dramatherapist at the University of Hertfordshire. He worked in the NHS for a number of years as a dramatherapist with adults and children with disabilities. He currently works as a therapist for a private fostering agency and is completing a PhD in drama education and dramatherapy at the University of Warwick.

Phil Jones, Reader, Institute of Education, has held the posts of Director of Research, School of Education, Faculty of Education, Social Sciences and Law, University of Leeds and Visiting Professor at Concordia University, Montreal, has lectured from South Africa to Canada, from South Korea to Australia and published widely on childhood and the arts therapies. His books include *Rethinking Childhood* (Continuum 2009), *Rethinking Children's Rights* (with Welch, Continuum 2010), *The Arts Therapies* (Routledge 2005), *Drama as Therapy* (Routledge 2007, 2010), *Childhood: Services and Provision* (with Moss, Tomlinson and

Welch, Pearson 2007), *Children's Rights in Practice* (with Walker, Sage 2011) and he is series editor for Continuum's *New Childhoods*.

Alison Kelly, dramatherapist and supervisor, works within the NHS and as a lecturer at Central School of Speech and Drama on the MA Drama and Movement Therapy (Sesame) training and she has a private therapy and supervision practice. With dramatherapist Alyson Coleman she co-runs Willow, a children's bereavement service for children who have life-limiting conditions within the NHS.

Catherine Kelly is a lecturer in educational and child psychology at the University of Manchester and a senior educational psychologist with Bury Educational Psychology Service. She has worked as a teacher and educational psychologist in local authorities in London, the South East and the North West, as well as a professional and academic tutor for the doctorate programme in education and child psychology at UCL. Her research interests include resilience and attributions, looked after children, group problem solving, and children and young people's participation.

Lauraine Leigh is a Health Professions Council Registered dramatherapist/psychotherapist and a teacher. After dramatherapy training at Hertfordshire University, she worked in Barnet, Waltham Forest, Reading and Slough schools. She has worked for 20 years in schools, pupil referral units, and with adolescents in hospitals. She is a member of the Tavistock and Portman NHS Trust, divides her work between Newbury, Henley and East London where she works with families and eating difficulties (www.familytherapy.co.uk and stoptellingmetoeat.co.uk). She offers INSET, meditation and training courses in Europe.

Olivia Lousada started as a Montessori teacher, then a secondary school teacher, before training in group work and social work. Grandparented as a dramatherapist, she is a senior trainer of psychodrama, working with a wide variety of people in psychiatric hospitals and education for over 30 years. She is a founder member of the London Psychodrama Network. Her doctorate and a book, *Hidden Twins. What Adult Opposite Sex Twins Have To Teach Us* (Karnac 2009) have resulted in her re-commitment to the importance of spontaneity and creativity in social, psychological and educational learning.

Brenda Meldrum is a state-registered arts therapist and play therapist. She runs Playing Matters, her company which trains therapists, counsellors and school staff to give emotional support to children and young people. Trained as a psychologist, Brenda takes an empirical as well as a playful approach to her work as a dramatherapist in a mainstream primary school in south London.

Daniel Mercieca works as a dramatherapist in Malta and specialises in work with children, adolescents and families facing emotional and behavioural difficulties, especially in out-of-home placements. He coordinates a transdisciplinary therapeutic team that works in the context of out-of-home care. He also trained in Applied Systemic Theory and Integrative Relational Supervision, and is one of the founding members of the Creative Arts Therapies Society in Malta.

Josephine Roger works as a dramatherapist and child psychotherapist in a primary school for children with severe and profound learning disabilities. She formerly worked as a teacher. She co-organised the first Dramatherapy in Education Now conference in 2000.

Deborah E. Shine currently works as a dramatherapist within a Devon primary school. She has worked within a range of settings, including education, mental health and residential care. Her practice is informed by the transference process. Having worked extensively with children and young people in social and secure care, Deborah has a particular interest in working therapeutically with attachment issues.

Carla Stavrou works as an educational psychologist in Cambridgeshire. She formerly worked as a secondary school English and drama teacher.

Matthew Trustman is a dramatherapist and senior lecturer in the psychological therapies department at Roehampton University, where he teaches on the Masters Dramatherapy and Dance and Movement Therapy programmes. An experienced teacher, facilitator, visual researcher and dramatherapist, he has a background in business management and management consultancy, and worked for the last seven years as a dramatherapist with school management teams, secondary schools pupils, their families and teachers.

Foreword

> You must be the change you wish to see in the world
>
> Mohandas K. Ghandi

This book has been a long time coming.

At a time when many dramatherapists are working in the education system, it is important to have a voice to speak out about what dramatherapists are doing. The editors and I hope this book encourages collaborative work, a sharing of paradigms and a willingness to see through a kaleidoscope of lenses, bringing into focus the gap between all of us who work with children in school settings.

Those of us working in schools hope this book provides an integrated understanding of the rationale underpinning the work of dramatherapists and hope that it will enable us to see our humble part in the greater whole, enhancing empathy and rapport within the wider school community and creating a fertile ground for mutual trust, respect and understanding to breed.

I hope this significant book will bring a sense of well-earned confidence among the community of dramatherapists working in education, as well as the staff who welcome this community into the safety of their school environment. Dramatherapists usually see the child, a group of children or a family under a clinical setting in schools. By doing so, dramatherapists can contain and support the teachers in what teachers are skilled to do: teaching.

The writers share one common and vital purpose with readers: our passion and care for the wellbeing of children and young people. Childhood is golden. Most of us have a deep knowing of the repercussions of a lost and damaged childhood. The signs of that are visible for all of us to see in the corridors and classrooms of schools.

My hope is that this book enables us to find a collective language to realize the inevitable vision of schools being the hub of interagency work which has the child at its centre.

Dimpi Hirani
Chair of The British Association of Dramatherapists in Education Sub Committee
January 2011

Preface

We would like to say a little about the reason for us wanting to produce this book, its genesis and underpinning thesis, and what we hope the book will achieve.

The book's genesis developed after Lauraine Leigh met Irvine Gersch. She had been working for several years, with the keen support of headteachers, in London secondary schools. As Principal Educational Psychologist in a London borough, Irvine was interested to hear about dramatherapy. He went on to give the keynote address for the first Dramatherapy in Education Now Conference in London in 2000. The initial connection between the two professions was tied.

In 2007 the editorial team grew and flourished with the addition of Ann Dix. Her experience working with a northern team in an area of multiple deprivation contributed greatly. Deborah Haythorne joining latterly as co-director of Roundabout, the largest dramatherapy charity, which has grown exponentially in 25 years in London, brought skills and insight and recent exciting research. Ideas evolved, helpfully stimulated by careful, detailed questioning by our publishers. We felt we had some important messages to clarify and disseminate to professionals in the world of education and mental health. Indeed, our intention was to make firm links across this spectrum.

Firstly, we believe that dramatherapy practice is not as well known as it could or should be in schools, nor is it a provision widely enough used in education or with children and young people. Research and experience by educational psychologists supports this view (e.g. Gersch, 2001; Gersch and Goncalves, 2006). Other evidence for this belief comes from informal, consistent reports from headteachers, school staff, local authority staff, young people, children, parents and dramatherapists themselves.

Secondly, we believe that dramatherapy has a great deal to offer, therefore a major part of this book is devoted to case studies. A section devoted to evidence and outcomes enables readers to make up their own minds about efficacy. Evaluation studies at the time of writing are 'work in progress', and they are impressive.

Thirdly, the editors believe that to maximize the effect of dramatherapy in schools, consideration should be given to the context, partnerships, and working with others. Sensitive planning, careful arrangements, procedures and communication are needed between dramatherapists and school staff. Learning from each other, bringing both different and complementary views about boundaries, expectations and rules to the table is a healthy process, as the chapter on 'Staff sharing' by Kelly and Bruck exemplifies.

We believe dramatherapy is under-used, an insufficiently tapped resource. It is ready to be further utilized, alongside the existing help for children. Gersch and Goncalves (2006) give convincing reasons why educational psychologists and dramatherapists can combine their forces to this end. Given the changing world in education, and the growth of choices open to schools, this is a timely point to make. Part V of the book, therefore, is devoted to some future possibilities and models for consideration, which add to this debate.

Practical as well as theoretical aspirations draw on the whole multi-disciplinary team working around the child, from the Educational Psychology Service to Child and Adolescent Mental Health Services (CAMHS). It is a salient feature of this book that dramatherapy is featured across the spectrum of children's mental health, from working preventatively with emotional wellbeing at one end, to working 1:1 and with families where there is very challenging behaviour and/or mental health diagnosis at the other.

The four chapters in the Introduction set the scene by discussing the role and relevance and nature of dramatherapy, written by three of the editors joined by Dokter, leading practitioner, author and academic. Her section on supervision has useful implications. The differences and similarities of dramatherapy and drama teaching are discussed by Holmwood and Stavrou. A stringent overview of the implications of dramatherapy in schools is provided by Reader in Childhood, international lecturer, Phil Jones. Meldrum, director of children's charity Playing Matters, cogently argues for adults to support children, drawing on Bowlby's work on attachment.

Case studies in part II comprise vivid examples by highly experienced practitioners. Dix details sensitive, creative work with a boy diagnosed with attention deficit hyperactivity disorder, now more commonly diagnosed than ever before. Dix also writes poignantly about her work with a sexually abused child, using the story of Red Riding Hood. Shine details effective short-term dramatherapy utilizing a neuroscientific input for a boy who miserably feared Math; Domikles, with a CAMHS background, engages an angry young man on the verge of exclusion. This has wide implications. Dooman's chapter movingly details skilful work with bereaved families. Carr meets urgent emotional needs through uniquely appropriate Shakespeare; Court, Higley and Lousada explain the enchanting draw of The Magic Shop. This suggests a template for today. Coleman and Kelly's work accompanies children through the unpredictable nature of illness and grief.

Part III of the book is devoted to collaborative partnerships in schools and beyond, given the critical importance of this complex issue in ensuring that dramatherapy is maximally effective in the service of the child. Roger's eloquent chapter is touching, salutary and also, wryly humorous. Kelly and Bruck implement their popular Staff Sharing model. Mercieca's hermeneutic, non-interventionist approach enables an unexpected shift for a mother moved by her son's sudden maturity. Trustman's film *Spare Me The Cutter* proves an ideal stimulus for the complex issue of safe working with self-harm. Clinical psychologist Brown, practising psychoanalytically based dramatherapy in France, identifies the power of the voice offstage. Haythorne details how Roundabout developed an impressive and growing popularity in London schools.

Part IV features positive evidence and outcomes. Educational psychologist Jennifer Greene reports parents see positive change in children's empathy and problem behaviour. Haythorne, Crockford and Godfrey focus on children's evaluations using Psychlops Kids: 'It was the best group I ever joined'. Madeline Andersen-Warren, recent chairperson of The British Association of Dramatherapists, cites BADth research: dramatherapy in schools is a growing field producing positive outcomes. Headteachers comment: 'Both parents and teachers are often forced to use a reward system to achieve cooperation. What dramatherapy did was to achieve this cooperation on a voluntary basis.'

Part V outlines future exciting potential and possibilities for schools, taking forward both therapeutic methodology and integrative, combined professional work. Irvine Gersch's research on listening to children is interesting and these children's comments sometimes profound. Listening adults support children, as does Meldrum's comprehensive model for primary schools. Lauraine Leigh's Dovetail model focuses on linking attachment patterns and the learning process in family dramatherapy. Finally, Rex Haigh, leader in the field in personality disorder and therapeutic communities, makes important points about non-verbal interventions and mental health.

The reader is led to reflect government spending on dramatherapy for schools must be an economical way forward. Irvine Gersch, Professor of Educational and Child Psychology at the University of East London, writes the decisive conclusion. As this book goes to press, new opportunities will enable positive links for schools wishing to develop wellbeing curricula.

This book is intended as a comprehensive resource for teachers, decision makers, policy makers, dramatherapy practitioners, aspiring dramatherapists, educational psychologists and their students, researchers, young people, allied professionals, sister arts therapists, actors, dramatists/drama lecturers, child psychiatrists and psychotherapists, clinical psychologists, school nurses and other mental health professionals. A book to dip into and to drink deeply from, its aim is to stimulate further research and greater use of this most exciting profession.

REFERENCES

Gersch, I.S. (2001) 'Dramatherapy in education: opportunities for the future — a view from the outside', *Dramatherapy, Special 'Education' Edition*, 23(1), 4–8.

Gersch, I.S. and Sao Joao Goncalves, S. (2006) 'Creative arts and educational psychology: let's get together', *International Journal of Art Therapy*, 11(1), 22–32.

Leigh, L. (2007) Thinking about a passion for truth: does drama, dramatherapy and psychoanalytic thinking have anything to offer schools? MA Dissertation, Tavistock and University of East London.

Acknowledgements

Lauraine Leigh would like to warmly thank Ann Dix, Deborah Haythorne and Irvine Gersch for invaluable colleagueship on steering this boat, and the chapter contributors: a great crew. To thank with love, Bek, Joe and Bud Leigh for their longtime support and patience, and also particularly Dr Carolyn Fraser for her helpful clarity in the editing process. Ann Dix would especially like to mention and thank for their love, patience and support Nick Daisley and Natalie Dix. Thanks for their abiding interest and encouragement to Mike Sharp, Angela Dougal, Cath Fraser, Freda Henderson, Maggie Jamieson, Patrick and Barbara Cogswell, Jean Tilbrook, and Jane Read particularly for incisive editing.

The Editors would like to thank their families for their support throughout the process of this book during its long gestation. Special thanks go to Barbara Gersch, who carried out careful proof reading and reviews of chapters at several stages of development, and whose patience and attention to detail is so much appreciated. Special thanks go to all the team at Roundabout.

We would like to thank our publishers Joanne Forshaw and Jane Harris and the team at Routledge for their invaluable guidance, support and advice.

Thanks to: The United Nations, Publications Board, New York, for their kind permission to cite sections from the United Nations Convention of the Child, Article 12, in Chapter 22, page 219, by Irvine Gersch; and *The British Association of Dramatherapists' Journal* for granting permission for the extract from 'Bringing learning disabilities into play within an educational setting' by Josephine Roger (*BADth Journal* Vol 23. Spring 2001).

Thanks too for generous interest to so many others, including: Adam Phillips, Susie Orbach, Hristo Georgiev for IT and especially Sydney Klugman and Annie Tunnicliffe. To Ruth Woodward, Dr Alex Horne and Val Haynes particularly, and to Dimpi Hirani, Claire Donnelly, Heidi Jokelson, Holly Harbour, Karen Kilberg, Holly Dwyer Hall, Emma Ramsden, Pauline Dutch. For valued colleagueship to Josephine Roger, Phil Jones and Sue Jennings. Mary Wellman, Tamara Collinson, Ruth

Goodman, Dan Burningham, Anna Chesner, Joan Crawford, Olivia Lousada, Mary Wellman, Maggie McAlister, Jean Taylor and Caroline Sanders. Professors Michael Rustin and Sue Rendall, Drs Amit Biswas, Ghazala Afzal and Rafiq Reefat, valued colleagues; Simon Wilkinson; Goffrey Court, Mary-Jayne Rust, Hilary Prentice, David Kennard, Carmel Conn, Angela Brinkworth, Anne Marie John, Mary Steel and Deborah Lacey. To Alida Gersie, warm thanks for setting the ball rolling. . .

Very special appreciation and thanks to the children, young people, teachers, professional colleagues and parents represented in case studies and vignettes, who have taught us so much.

The views and ideas expressed in the chapters within this book remain those of the writers alone. They do not necessarily reflect those of other contributors to the book, the editorial team, or any of their respective employers.

Thanks to Linda Laletin for her valued contribution to Chapter 1.

Part I

Introduction

1 The role and relevance of dramatherapy in schools today

Lauraine Leigh, Ann Dix, Ditty Dokter and Deborah Haythorne

Introduction

Why should schools need dramatherapy?

There is something of a revolution taking place in education today. Schools are faced with the choice of opting out of local authority control to become Academies or Free Schools. For those that remain with the local authority there are further changes to the curriculum. Support services may be cut and finances refocused, leaving schools to manage the emotional wellbeing of the children they teach. There is a shift in thinking, which suggests that emotional health should become a part of the school's responsibility, yet teachers, already under pressure to teach, will find this a challenge.

Just how much we should be concerned about children's mental health is indicated by the November 2010 Scottish Integrative Care Programme for Child and Adolescent Mental Health Services (CAMHS): 'Mental health problems in children and young people are more common than many realise'. The Public Health Institute for Scotland Needs Assessment Report on CAMHS (2003: 3) states that about 10% of children and young people 'have mental health problems which are so substantial that they have difficulties with their thoughts, their feelings, their behaviour, their learning, their relationships, on a day-to-day basis'. Children's behaviour can become problematic as they try to make sense of their chaotic lives, and this obviously has a big impact on schools and the wider community.

Dramatherapists have been working effectively in schools for over twenty years and this book suggests an even greater need for dramatherapy in schools. The role of the dramatherapist can be to bridge the gap between education and mental health, working in schools alongside and in tandem with teachers and other professional staff, with the child and young person at the centre. An understanding of the use of therapy in schools has evolved, even though parents and children may still struggle with a fear of stigmatization (Carr and Ramsden 2008). Many parents and adolescents actively request dramatherapy. The provision of help through dramatherapy towards supporting good mental health in children and young people within schools can depathologize the problems children and young people experience, and make it a part of normal development. There is significant evidence that dramatherapy is effective in working with children in schools (see part IV).

Who are dramatherapists?

Dramatherapists come from many walks of life including teaching, nursing and mental health professions such as clinical psychology, primary mental health workers, and from arts and theatre related professions. A large percentage of dramatherapists work in educational settings with children and young people. Some are employed by the local authority, or directly by the school. Many work freelance, building up a network of relationships within the school community. Some work for CAMHS and other agencies that provide therapeutic support to schools. Many dramatherapists work for charities such as Roundabout and The Place2B.

What is dramatherapy?

The British Association of Dramatherapists (BADth) offers the following definition of dramatherapy:

> Dramatherapy has as its main focus the intentional use of the healing aspects of drama and theatre within the therapeutic process. It is a method of working and playing which uses action to facilitate creativity, imagination, learning, insight, and growth.

It is mandatory for all dramatherapists to be registered with The Health Professions Council whose Standards of Proficiency for Arts Therapists document (2007) describes dramatherapy as:

> a unique form of psychotherapy in which creativity, play, movement, voice, storytelling, dramatisation, and the performance arts have a central position within the therapeutic relationship.

As this book demonstrates, dramatherapy sessions may use a wide selection of techniques to engage the child or young person, individually or in groups in schools. These include cooperative games, story telling, drawing and painting and the use of materials to create stories and plays. This metaphorical work can be non-verbal or verbal, using speech, script and/or movement. Jenkyns' work with adults would suggest exciting possibilities for adolescents and children, utilizing published texts (Jenkyns 1996), and indeed, Carr writes of her work in an inner city school using Shakespearian text with adolescents (chapter 9). Dramatherapy uses metaphor, to enable the child to begin to express their feelings safely and to feel better about themselves. The use of 'as if' allows dramatic distance so that the child is not overwhelmed or re-traumatized.

Each session will be planned to allow the child to work at their own pace and children and young people are not required to talk about their difficulties if they are not comfortable doing so. By creating a safe therapeutic space the dramatherapist sets the scene and waits for the child to begin to move centre stage.

Dramatherapy in schools

Difficult behaviour in classrooms

Difficult behaviour in classrooms can indicate emotional difficulties at home; for instance, the separation of parents or the death of a grandparent. Children who are feeling vulnerable can become less tolerant of schoolmates and they may have difficulty in settling in lessons, deliberately flout rules and may constantly challenge teachers, verbally and physically. Domikles (chapter 7) makes the point that sometimes difficult behaviour is a symptom of mental health issues. If these can be diagnosed funding for mental health interventions may be offered to schools. There is a clear link, then, between challenging behaviour in schools as an indicator of young people's anxieties, and mental health issues which become visible in adolescence and are later diagnosed in adolescence and adulthood. Leading psychoanalyst Margot Waddell (2005) refers to adolescence as 'a narcissistic disorder' and suggests that for some young people the impact of puberty is a 'kind of detonation' which they can spend the rest of their lives getting used to. This impacts on their relationship with the world and on their ability to cope with adulthood (L. Leigh: personal record of Margot Waddell's address to the Institute of Psychoanalysis: November 2005).

Dramatherapists in schools notice that peer pressure exerts a strong influence on children and it would appear that growing numbers of children feel the need to join the periphery of difficult behaviour. There are many reasons for this, including boredom, to be 'acceptable' to their peers, or to challenge authority. Of significant and growing concern to parents and teachers is gang membership and violent behaviour.

Bullying in and out of school can be subtle or overt and the rise of social networking sites makes this more difficult to monitor. Schools are therefore key in helping. This is an issue of education. Anti-bullying issues are high on school agendas. These issues can be addressed by teachers, dramatherapists and educational psychologists, and Holmwood and Stavrou (chapter 3) examine how dramatherapists and drama teachers might work alongside the educational psychology profession in integrative ways to promote ways of working with drama for just these sorts of issues.

Dramatherapy provides an ideal medium to explore difficult, painful issues, to build resilience in children and young people. Group work can provide a reflective space for children to confront their prejudices and fears.

Working with children who are diagnosed and working with those who are not

In schools dramatherapists work with a wide range of children and young people, including those who have emotional and behavioural problems, children who have experienced abuse, trauma, bereavement and loss, and those who experience discrimination such as refugees and asylum seekers or children in the care system. Children with diagnosed mental health issues such as severe anxiety, attention deficit hyperactivity disorder (ADHD), oppositional defiant disorder (ODD), or conduct disorder (CD), and autistic spectrum disorder (ASD) make up a large percentage of our client group, together with children who have learning difficulties, and children who get into conflict in school. In this book we include vignettes of work with children and young people of all ages and abilities, ethnicities and cultures. We respect different cultural and religious values, and it is central to our profession that we work to foster tolerance.

Working together

The British Association of Dramatherapists have a helpful website that includes information about dramatherapy in schools, highlighting the areas in which dramatherapists can offer their services, including staff training, diagnostic assessments and short- and long-term dramatherapy interventions. Dramatherapists work according to the BADth Code of Ethical Practice. Central to dramatherapy practice are consent, safeguarding, liaison, health and safety and continuing professional development.

Dramatherapists work throughout the education system, working closely with teachers, parents, educational psychologists (EPs), CAMHS, social care, psychiatrists, and other agencies through the child assessment frameworks (CAF), the courts and reviews.

Supervision supports safe practice and offers a place for dramatherapists to reflect on their work. Later in this chapter Dokter, leading dramatherapy practitioner and academic, describes the importance of supervision for dramatherapists. As Dokter and the supervisees who have provided the vignettes highlight, there are implications for the teaching profession, because nowadays particularly, teachers also need emotional support in their work. Kelly and Bruck (chapter 14) put forward an effective, evaluated model of integrative staff support.

It is the responsibility of parents and professionals to ensure positive outcomes for children and young people. In order to support the child, their teachers, parents and carers also need support, so that the child's needs can be addressed systemically. Many dramatherapists include family therapy in their continuous professional development, recognizing the need for a systemic approach to their work. 'No man is an island' and the most effective way of helping the child is by supporting their family network where possible. 'Families' voices have moved centre stage such that some therapists regard therapy as essentially the process of conversing, of engaging in storytelling and making' (Dallos and Draper 2000: 11). The teacher, paediatrician and psychoanalyst Winnicott made the point, 'When we are able to help parents to help their children we do in fact help them about themselves' (2003 [1958]: 308).

Boundaries and working agreements

The use of simple, effective boundaries and the opportunity to discuss them is an important part of any dramatherapy session. Boundaries such as 'No put-downs' and 'You can say "Pass"' hold a useful appeal for children and young people, giving them a sense of ownership and control as well as a feeling of safety. The work's non-judgemental ethos for children and teenagers appears to be easily understood by most young people, including children new to the UK, possibly with limited English language. These boundaries have the advantage of being accessible, easily remembered, and acceptable. Luxmoore's *Feeling Like Crap* (2008) describes the attitudes that can so easily be prevalent for teenagers in their search for identity. This boundary making is a most important foundation for those with continuing challenging behaviour, who may have little patience for going through a set of rules posted on a wall.

However, some children and young people do respond well to setting up a 'working agreement' at the beginning of a dramatherapy intervention that can be discussed and agreed verbally or may be presented as a written and signed document. The first part of the agreement is to explain and discuss consent with regards to the children and young people attending dramatherapy and to discuss confidentiality. The rest of the agreement focuses on the rules of the group and is usually worked out between the children and young people and the therapists.

Therapy takes place within school and therefore, although there may be boundaries or rules within the session, school rules need to be adhered to and the child needs to be aware of this. The child needs to return to class in a composed and settled manner. Dramatherapy with its emphasis on the concept of 'de-rolement', means that attention is always paid to de-roling and relaxation at the end of the session.

The teacher–therapist partnership is key

Confidentiality is also an important factor in the provision of dramatherapy. Good relationships between teachers and dramatherapists ensure the work of each is respected: Roger (chapter 13) details the importance of the ongoing and effective communication between dramatherapist and teacher who talk together regularly about the young people. She highlights how this partnership of adults is key to affecting the young people's own feelings of safety in dramatherapy, and therefore its effectiveness. The dramatherapist communicates with the teacher as well as keeping the confidentiality of sessions. Confidentiality in the dramatherapy sessions is explained to the children and young people within the context of safeguarding, recognizing that there are times when other appropriate named adults may need to know about what has been shared in a session.

Models of dramatherapy

Reference is made in this book to a variety of models of dramatherapy, some well established, including Jennings' EPR developmental model (chapters 5 and 24) and Read Johnson's DvT model. Domikles (chapter 7) offers an adaptation of the latter, working as a primary mental health worker. Shine highlights the outstanding effectiveness of her short-term neuroscientific dramatherapy model (chapter 6); Coleman and Kelly (chapter 12) have developed an impressive systemic model for working with children with life-limiting conditions, and working with their siblings before and after the child's death. Brown's model for autistic and psychotic children appears to enable excitingly an inner distinction for these children between reality and play on a stage (chapter 17). Trustman describes the dramatherapist and teacher working together with the whole class on the issue of self-harm (chapter 16); Court, Higley and Lousada as teachers, artist in residence and psychodramatist (chapter 11), combined their variety of sensitive and skillful approaches with whole classes.

Adults working together to support the child or young person is a feature of this book. There is an exploration of how sharing ideas and information can be useful for educational psychologists, dramatherapists and teachers in Kelly and Bruck's chapter 14. Encouraging parents into school to support their child is vital, is often hard work, and the Dovetail model (chapter 24) combines psychoanalytical concepts with Jennings' EPR developmental model in the service of this aim. The work by the two London-based charities, Roundabout (chapter 18) and Playing Matters (chapter 23) is impressively and clearly described. Playing Matters trains adults to communicate effectively with children and young people. Roundabout is the largest service provider of dramatherapy in schools in the UK and works closely with teaching staff. Roundabout's recent positive evaluation of dramatherapy in schools is essential reading (chapter 19).

Assessment and outcomes

Dramatherapists sometimes use the 6 Part Story Method (6PSM) for children and young people in schools, as an indicator of their preoccupations.

Whether or not the behaviour and needs of these young people in schools is diagnosable or diagnosed (which entails close work with CAMHS), Kim Dent Brown's 6PSM, which acknowledges the work of Mooli Lahad and Alida Gersie, offers both a useful assessment tool and a simple springboard for story making and drama.

It is of no little significance that this assessment is used increasingly in the NHS as a predictor of borderline personality disorder with adults (Dent-Brown and Wang 2004).

Dramatherapy work is evaluated in a number of different ways, including using the 'Strengths and Difficulties Questionnaire' (SDQ), Goodman et al. (1998), PSYCHLOPS Kids (chapter 19) and the Health of the Nation Outcome Scales for Children and Adolescents (HoNOSCA; Gowers et al. 1999). Later chapters in this book discuss impressive evaluation (chapters 19, 20 and 21). Dramatherapists often create their own user-led evaluation forms which feature behaviour and social development. The Leigh Evaluation form (developed in 1999; Leigh, personal communication) uses teachers' observations about the child before, during and after work looking at a range of issues including learning skills, cooperation and communication with peers,

Teachers' evaluations of dramatherapy **Date............**

To .... Class/Subject teacher of ....

Child's name................................... Class/Form...................................

It would help us both to see a rounded picture of how useful dramatherapy is if you could kindly take 2 minutes to tick and evaluate any change or not in this child's abilities in the classroom, after 6/8/10 weeks/1 term/2 terms/ 1 academic year of dramatherapy. Positives will be discussed in dramatherapy with the child. This form will be compared with a final evaluation after the final session.
Thank you for your time..................................Dramatherapist

	Significantly poorer	Poorer	No change	Improvement	Significant improvement	Any comment
Listening skills						
Speaking skills						
Cooperation with peers						
Cooperation with teacher						
Communication with teacher						
Communication with peers						

Please add any other comment overleaf. Date returned to dramatherapist.............

Figure 1.1 Teachers' evaluation form

other children and teachers. Designed to be completed in two minutes, this evaluation includes a five-point negative to positive scale, similar to Likert (chapter 20), which simply requires a tick. Alongside this and overleaf the teacher can comment briefly (see Figure 1).

Measurable outcomes are important in assessing the value of dramatherapy. The individual recorded responses from parents, teachers and pupils below are equally valid.

Dramatherapists use a variety of evaluation forms to capture this information and below is a selection of comments from around the country.

Parents

> The therapists are not only great fun, showing an amazing understanding of the children in their care, but are incredibly approachable and have given me as a parent enormous support.

> . . .it is the dramatherapy that has helped him the most. It gives him confidence, which he has always lacked, and helps with his imagination. It was something for him to look forward to and helped him to develop relationships at school.

> As a child with 'ASD' my child constantly struggles to cope with change. The dramatherapy team have helped him bring out his true self.

> I felt a weight lifted.

Teachers

> They (the dramatherapists) freely give feedback and have been a tremendous source of help and encouragement.

> I cannot praise the dramatherapy service more highly and wish we had more funding so they could be on site more than once a week.

> He has enjoyed his time on the dramatherapy sessions more than I expected. He has benefited from being able to express himself in a setting where he feels totally included. This child is a very creative and a visual learner, so attending the sessions has enabled him to express himself even more.

Pupils and students

> Dramatherapy has helped me to calm down and not to fight with other people when they're interested in fighting.

> Dramatherapy made me feel happy.

Now I am not so worried about my new school.

I felt stronger about going back into Y9 class after dramatherapy.

Dokter writes on supervision

Dramatherapists do not work alone. As with all recognized psychotherapies, the support around the therapist is vital to the support they themselves offer. External supervision plays a vital role in supporting the dramatherapist at all times, particularly working in schools. Clinical supervision of dramatherapy has become a well-established practice over the last 25 years (Dokter 2008) and it is a mandatory part of the training.

This raises an important question. The teaching profession does not integrally receive supervision, which is often seen as a part of performance management. *Unless there is a separation of the managerial supervision, which provides support and guidance, and the separate clinical supervision, which allows a space to reflect on the emotional effects of working with children, there will always be a conflict of interest.* One way of working with this problem is to have joint supervision sessions between therapists and teachers in order to foster a common language and understanding.

The following vignette is written by a teacher who is also a dramatherapist. The vignette illustrates the role of supervision in containing the teacher/therapist development.

Supervision vignette 1

My first dramatherapy post was in a special school in which I had been a teacher for eight years. I worked as a dramatherapist in Key Stage 3 and 4 and continued to teach drama part time in the post-16 department.

After 20 years as a teacher, becoming a dramatherapist required a different way of thinking about working with children. As a therapist, I felt very isolated in the workplace. Surrounded by teaching colleagues, it was easy to continue to think from a behavioural perspective. Supervision continued to be essential to help me reflect on children from a therapeutic stance. Some teachers put in place their strict behavioural contracts with pupils, which may have to an extent dealt with behaviours, but these did not get to the heart of helping the child. Supervision helped to develop my confidence so that in my role of dramatherapist I could encourage staff to look a bit deeper, to empathize with the child and to consider supportive strategies.

Supervision helped me to find ways to strengthen my own boundaries and care for myself. I needed to, because the children's lives were overwhelmingly difficult. This included accepting what I could not change as well as reflecting on what support I could reasonably give. Whilst I could not rescue the children, I could help them build their

> resilience. It became clear that working with parents and helping them to understand their child and make changes to support their child was an important part of my role. Some parents were resistant to reflecting on their own way of being with their children; the important thing is to empathise with them. As with my child clients, supervision helped me to develop empathy for parents. The use of role play in supervision gave me insight into the parents' perspective, and enabled me to prepare for potentially sensitive parent meetings.
>
> Supervision has given me confidence as well as being able to understand my limitations. For instance I am now able to confidently advocate for children when speaking with head teachers, teachers, parents, social workers etc. I also have the confidence to accept and state limitations of my work. Now I can process my feelings of inadequacy. Supervision has helped me to develop my own internal supervisor.

Carr and Ramsden (2008) also describe the potential benefits for teachers of receiving dramatherapy supervision. One of the areas of benefit is that of understanding diversity and difference. Dramatherapy treatment can support development for marginalized groups and as such meet many of the recommendations for good practice around equality and diversity for marginalized groups (NICE 2010).

The second vignette focuses on an after-school intervention for primary school children referred by social services and their teachers for being at risk of exclusion. Some experienced learning difficulties and behavioural problems.

In a rural setting, an after-school group intervention was chosen to enable access. The dramatherapy aim was greater integration into the school community, exploration of difficulties around bullying and exclusion, and working on areas of conflict within the children's families. The practice supervised has been published in Department of Health examples of good practice (Department of Health 2008).

Supervision vignette 2

Brief overview of after-school dramatherapy

To set up and provide 14 sessions of a community dramatherapy group for children.

Group 1 was with 8 children. The location was in a children's centre adjacent to the school.

Group 2 was with 9 children. The location was in a children's centre inside the school.

Some main issues

Group 1: Two of the group members were cousins. One of the group members was living with a parent who is suffering with mental illness. All children experienced learning difficulties in their mainstream school. The main themes were depression and deprivation.

Group 2: Eight children attended the same school, one child attended a different school. Four of the group members were in single-parent families, two group members were twins. Two group members have had or are currently receiving statutory social work support and intervention. Fifty percent of group members are from low-income households, all have mixed cognitive abilities.

How clinical supervision supported group management and context

The supervision discussed the structuring and form for the groups. This enabled reflective space to see the individuals in each group and also their way of interacting with each other. This mirrored the intentions of the dramatherapist and helped give meanings to interventions used.

One of the difficulties was establishing boundaries for both groups. Many of the group members exhibited behavioural difficulties, which could result in scapegoating and bullying within the group dynamics. This also occurred in the school and contributed to the children's marginalization, so it was crucial to find ways of addressing and working with these dynamics.

> In Group 1 the children wanted to play with preschool toys. In this group, where depression was a theme, small world work (Jones 2007) was utilized. The play with objects expanded to showing and doing through role-play and embodiment.
>
> In Group 2 I found myself running around the group of children as if I were a sheep dog. The group struggled to accept authority, which had led to conflict in the classroom with teachers. They were also very competitive and found it hard to work together. I encouraged the children to make agreements on 'self rule' alongside negotiating agreements with myself and my co-worker.
>
> Family constellation work acknowledged who knew who and who was connected to whom. This 'owning' enabled both groups to settle into an equitable hierarchy.
>
> Clinical supervision ensured that I paid particular attention to my interpersonal style as well as the co-working relationship. Psychodynamic understanding of the clients' relationship difficulties being contained and worked through by the co-workers meant that it was important to firm up our own respective responsibilities, alongside our emotional reactions to the individual's behaviour and group dynamics.

This informs the parallel process of what is going on within the group and for the facilitators.

This parallel process is one of the areas of focus for supervision (Dokter 2008; Carr and Ramsden 2008). I further used my clinical supervision for consultation, advice, support, seeking to review and monitor the progress of each individual child. Each child's progress was monitored through the SCOPE (Model of Human Occupation Theory and Application; Kielhofner 2008) outcome measure. Clinical supervision supported the intention, meaning and purpose of the project. It felt like the groups became a shared ownership; the therapeutic work was not being done in isolation. I was not alone.

The above two vignettes support:

- the therapeutic containment of the client
- the focus of process and outcomes of the therapy for the child/young person
- collaboration with teachers and parents
- professional development of the dramatherapist
- understanding of the organizational, family and individual client dynamics in the work.

Training as a dramatherapist

Currently dramatherapists train at MA level. There are five Health Professions Council (HPC) approved dramatherapy training courses in the UK. They are based in Cambridge, Derby, Exeter, London and Roehampton. These training courses take between 18 months and 3 years. Further contact details can be found in the websites section at the end of this book.

Conclusion

This chapter outlines some of the main policy and points of dramatherapists working in educational settings. It looks in detail at what supervision offers dramatherapists and why it is so much a part of their work. The implications are that teachers could benefit from similar emotional support. See also Kelly and Bruck (chapter 14), whose new model relates to skills sharing for teachers, educational psychologists and dramatherapists together.

Never before has there been such a need in schools for dramatherapists and other arts therapists, play therapists and creative therapists. This book shows the role of the dramatherapist is important in bridging the gap between education and mental health, working within schools in accepting, non-judgemental ways whilst also adhering to boundaries and school rules and listening to and essentially supporting teachers in their work. The aim of this work is largely preventive, which means children are less likely to go on to require the input of adult mental health services, thus reducing societal costs.

Finally, dramatherapy work in schools requires robustness and a continuous dialogue with head teachers, school staff and parents. This book contains details of emerging new dramatherapy models in schools, which require further research. As Karkou suggests in her recent book *Arts Therapies in Schools: Research and Practice*: 'one of the most important theoretical contributions . . . is to develop therapeutic models that are directly linked with school practice' (Karkou 2010: 275).

This chapter includes several testimonials about this work. The authors of this chapter make the point that that the role and relevance of dramatherapy in schools today appears to be essential in working preventively, helping maintain the mental health and wellbeing of children and young people within the learning environment.

Bibliography

BADth (2009) *Education sub-committee 'Dramatherapy in Education'*. Leaflet available from BADth. (See the helpful websites listed at the end of this book.)

BADth home page: http://www.badth.org.uk (accessed 23 January 2011).

Carr, M., and Ramsden, E. (2008) 'An exploration of supervision in education', in P. Jones and D. Dokter (eds.), *Supervision of Dramatherapy*. London: Routledge.

Child & Adolescent Mental Health Services (CAMHS) in NHS Scotland (2010) *Characteristics of the Workforce Supply*. http://www.isdscotland.org/isd/5379.html (accessed 24 January 2011).

Dallos, R., and Draper, R. (2000) *An Introduction to Family Therapy. Systemic Theory and Practice*. Milton Keynes: Open University Press.

Dent-Brown, K., and Wang, M. (2004) Developing a rating scale for projected stories. *Psychology and Psychotherapy. Theory, Research and Practice* 77: 325–333.

Department of Health (2008) *Good Practice for After School Groups*. http://www.ehow.co.uk/how_7739415_run-after-school-program.html (accessed 29 January 2011).

Dokter, D. (2008) 'Training supervision in dramatherapy', in P. Jones and D. Dokter (eds.), *Supervision of Dramatherapy*. London: Routledge.

DSM-IV-TR (2000) *Diagnostic and Statistical Manual of Mental Disorders*, fourth edition. Arlington, VA: American Psychiatric Association.

Goodman, R., Meltzer, H., and Bailey, V. (1998) 'The Strengths and Difficulties Questionnaire: A pilot study on the validity of the self-report version'. *European Child and Adolescent Psychiatry* 7: 125–130.

Gowers, S.G., Harrington, R.C., Whitton, A., Lelliott, P., Wing, J., Beevor, A., and Jezzard, R. (1999) 'A brief scale for measuring the outcomes of emotional and behavioural disorders in children: HoNOSCA'. *British Journal of Psychiatry* 174: 413–416.

Health Professions Council (2007) *Standards of Proficiency – Arts Therapists*. http://

www.hpc-uk.org/publications/standards/index.asp?id=39 (accessed 24 January 2011).

Jenkyns, M. (1996) *The Play's the Thing: Exploring Text in Drama and Therapy*. London: Routledge.

Jennings, S. (1990) *Dramatherapy with Families, Groups and Individuals. Waiting in the Wings*. London: Jessica Kingsley Publishers.

Karkou, V. (ed.) (2010) *Arts Therapies in Schools: Research and Practice*. London: Jessica Kingsley Publishers.

Kielhofner, G. (2008) *Model of Human Occupation Theory and Application*. 4th Ed. Baltimore: Lippincott Williams & Wilkins.

Luxmoore, N. (2008) *Feeling Like Crap*. London: Jessica Kingsley Publishers.

NICE (2010) *Guidelines on Equality*. http://www.nice.org.uk/media/953/E5/NICE'sEqualitySchemeActionPlan200710.pdf (accessed 29 January 2011).

Scottish Needs Assessment Programme (SNAP) (2003) *Report on Child – CAMHS*. http://www.handsonscotland.co.uk/publications/snap%20report.pdf (accessed 24 January 2011).

The Common Assessment Framework (DCSF) (2009) http://www.cwdcouncil.org.uk/caf (accessed 26 January 2011).

Waddell, M. (2005) *Adolescence: A Narcissistic Disorder*. Address to the Institute of Psychoanalysis, 25 November 2005. Personal record, Lauraine Leigh.

Winnicott, D.W. (1956) *The Anti-Social Tendency*. Reprinted in *Through Paediatrics to Psycho-analysis*, London: Hogarth Press, 1975.

Winnicott, D.W. (2003 [1958]) *From Paediatrics to Psychoanalysis. Collected Papers*. London: Karnac.

Winnicott, D.W. (1986) *Home Is Where We Start From. Essays by a Psychoanalyst*. London: Penguin Books.

2 Childhood today and the implications for dramatherapy in schools

Phil Jones

Introduction

The relationship between schools, education and therapy is complex and ambivalent: subject to changes made by shifts in cultural attitudes and politically driven policies. Should schools offer therapy to children? Should the school be a centre of excellence in curriculum-based subjects or a hub for multi-agency services to help them meet the needs of children and their families? Within the UK a part of this complexity is due to the particular route we have chosen for the provision of educational policies for our school system. From another perspective, the ambivalence about the identity and nature of schooling can be seen as cultural, and it relates to the ways in which a fragmentation of experience has been created whereby areas of children's lives such as health, education, social care, recreation and play have been separated out. In the UK we are so used to this way of segmenting our lives as children and adults, as users and providers of separated services, that it is often hard to see that this is a very *particular* way of living, working and providing. This chapter explores such fragmentation in the UK, the choices that have been made about the form and nature of education services such as schools, and their impact both on children and on the position of therapeutic services such as dramatherapy. It also looks at current developments that are challenging and changing traditional frameworks. In the early twenty-first century we are seeing changes in ideas about UK services for children. These changes come from a number of directions, but all are concerned, in one way or another, with this demarcation. This chapter will identify and critically examine these changes, which concern the emergence of initiatives that emphasize integration of services and interagency approaches to work with children. It looks critically at the contemporary situation and the changing face of ideas, practices and policies from a child rights and child-centred approach. These changes will be explored in relation to dramatherapy practice in schools.

Therapy and education: tensions and opportunities

Educational provision and its relationship to areas such as care, health and play have recently come under particular kinds of scrutiny and review (Wahidin and Moss 2004; Tomlinson 2008; Jones 2009a; Jones and Welch 2010). In considering the current situation in the UK, it can be useful to look at both the tensions we experience and the potentials for future innovation in the light of the way education and therapy provision have developed. A number of themes and issues have been identified that concern the nature of settings such as schools, and whether they serve or fail children (Rogers 2004; Tomlinson 2008). The terrible consequence of our approaches to practice and to structuring and funding services is illustrated in the ways in which children have suffered and been killed. One case that foregrounded the ways services can fail children, and that proved one of the key catalysts for recent change, was that of Victoria Climbié. Tomlinson draws attention to the 'high profile enquiry into the death of Victoria Climbié, responding to public and professional concerns about weaknesses in child protection strategy: children were once again on the government agenda' (2008: 29). She identifies the concern that children such as Victoria, 'a young child abused and finally murdered by her carers in spite of being brought to the attention of a range of welfare agencies' (2008: 29), was directly linked to a lack of connection between services. From the national review (Laming 2003) emerged an increasing recognition that processes such as the separation and division of services such as education, welfare and health were creating disturbing and fatal situations for children. One of the many implications of this has been an identified need to integrate services, and to move away from a cultural view of education and the school as a castle with walls constructed to keep concerns other than the national curriculum out. It has been accompanied by a reviewing of professional practice that creates ways of working that do not split off education from support services such as therapy provision. As Cross has said:

> The need for interagency and multidisciplinary working and co-operation involves many professionals. For example, with the concept of extended schools becoming more of a reality the class teacher's role in child health is increasingly key and is broadening beyond education in its traditional sense. It is often the teacher who notices if a child is unwell or experiencing difficulties and who refers this to the parents/guardians or others as necessary.
>
> (2008: 122)

Outside of the UK other models of living and working are in operation. Some have argued that there is a clear division between the English-speaking world, and models that have been created there, and those from other traditions. Moss, for example, contrasts the English approach, which has emphasized separation and division, as if there is no alternative, with that of Sweden, where integration of services for children, such as education and health,

> has been supported by re-thinking concepts of the child and of learning and by a well-established concept of pedagogy, which addresses children and young people holistically and aims to support their all round development. Reform of the Swedish workforce is also based on sustained and substantial public investment, which has led to the erosion of training and pay differentials between the professions whose training has now been integrated.
>
> (Moss 2003: 2)

Moss has pointed out that, despite the continuous, ongoing failures and shortcomings of the English-language cultured approach, and the comparative successes of others, the UK persists in chiefly looking to its traditional models and ignoring others.

As discussed above, in the late twentieth century it became clear that such a system of provision was failing children. Actions in the form of policy such as the Children Act (DfES 2004) and the Children's Plan engaged with such debates about whether settings such as schools could be changed to meet children and their families' capabilities and needs, and whether education needed to be reframed in the context of policies and practices that encouraged the multi-agency or the multidisciplinary. Such policies responded to the developing critique from disciplines such as the new sociology of childhood (Prout 2000; Archard and Macleod 2002; Jones and Welch 2010). One of the critiques is that the UK school system, in design or practice, does not serve children effectively. Such arguments assert that schools are primarily designed to serve adult needs or interests (Welch 2008). Critics have argued that UK education is still influenced by particular attitudes and discourses of childhood that see children as an investment, for example, and, whatever the overt veneer, that the system is primarily designed to turn children into adults who will well serve the national economy, or to satisfy other adult-orientated goals. In addition, critics have suggested that the move towards a target- and outcome-driven model in education has increasingly made schools a space in children's lives where they are continuously framed within a system that prioritizes the collection of specific kinds of outcome data. This, they argue, has resulted in a plethora of examinations, testing and surveillance at a level that is unprecedented (Bottery 1990; Welch 2008). Concerns have also been voiced that the lack of input from children in the design of provision means that models of schooling, even when they respond more widely to children's situations by providing support services, such as therapy, may not meet the real needs of children, but of those thought appropriate for them by adults' perceptions of children's states of mind or needs (Jones 2009a). If the child's voice is not sought or addressed, then the danger is that adult perceptions of provision are the only ones paid attention to, and that children's own perceptions of education, of a full, healthy life or of the need for therapy are not asked for, heard, or brought into the design of services in general, and therapeutic provision in particular.

The need for therapy in schools: multidisciplinarity and multi-agency working

Changes can be seen within the way UK policy is addressing issues in children's lives and the services they use. The emphasis is increasingly upon services that are designed for, and with, children, rather than designed to meet adults' agendas without any real consideration of children's actual needs. This is, naturally, an enormous task and is problematic, given the tensions within policies and the organizations they connect to. After decades of one system dominating, the changes we are beginning to hear about on paper, and in trial initiatives, demand major shifts in attitude, training, and practice in order to be successful. These tensions have been identified as:

- The outcome-driven culture of much education policy versus the more individualized child-centred approaches within some sectors of the school system.
- Attitudes of policy makers and organizations such as schools towards children, tending to view them as subjects rather than agents with valid ideas and opinions.
- Society-wide attitudes towards children as an investment rather than the seeing of childhood as a period of life with its own needs and demands.
- Training of those working with children that emphasizes individual specialisms rather than fostering interdisciplinary awareness.
- The need for resourcing that values the input of different professionals in children's lives within schools and that supports the necessary expenditure to develop quality rather than piecemeal lip-service provision.
- Policy that creates opportunities for schools to become genuine places for interagency use, rather than creating tensions over available time, for funding, and in satisfying contradictory government or local authority set aims and outcomes (Prout 2000; Archard and Macleod 2002; Jones 2009a; Jones and Welch 2010).

Every Child Matters (DfES 2003), the *National Services Framework for Children* (DoH 2005) and the *Children's Plan* (DfES 2007) were three examples of early twenty-first century UK policy developments with implications for therapy and children. The rhetoric of *Every Child Matters* promotes children's health; the *National Services Framework* oversees the development and implementation of a series of specific, targeted policy documents and initiatives. The *Children's Plan*, for example, seemed to acknowledge the need to support a widening of services to meet children's needs in areas that are allied to dramatherapy: those of play provision and mental health support. It committed to the creation of more playgrounds and a 'Play Strategy' along with a 'review' of Child and Adolescent Mental Health Services to 'see how universal, mainstream and specialist support services can be improved for the growing number of children and young people with mental health needs' (DfES 2007: 7). Critics have responded to initiatives such as the *Children's Plan* by identifying the ways in which tensions such as those outlined above may frustrate its aims. The NSPCC's immediate response to the *Children's Plan*, for example, reflects such critiques. NSPCC director and chief executive Dame Mary Marsh has argued that the *Children's Plan* forms an opportunity to improve outcomes for children. The NSPCC's position, as outlined by her, makes a clear warning and call for action: it is that children will simply not achieve their educational potential 'unless there are sufficient resources to address major problems such as violence, abuse and bullying' (NSPCC 2007). She situates a key element of this policy-driven initiative within interagency work and in developing practice to enable children to benefit from the combined value of professionals such as teachers and therapists making 'a positive difference to children'. She describes the policy as a 'blueprint' that services and professionals need to build upon to ensure that the plan is put into action through provision such as 'school counsellors and therapy for children who have been abused' (NSPCC 2007).

The NSPCC stressed the necessity of matching goals with adequate funding and directly identified the need not only for direct provision of therapeutic support, but for a financial commitment to training for other staff in areas such as the capacity to identify children who are in need of therapy, and to know how to refer them. The following gives an indication of their assessment of scale of this need:

> For every full double-decker school bus, seven children will be seriously unhappy and around three will be in fear of violence between their parents. Most of the lower deck will at some time during their childhood go home to serious worries. There must also be adequate training and support for professionals such as teachers, school nurses and youth workers to ensure they can recognise and respond to signs of abuse. The NSPCC has been calling on the Government to provide every school with a counsellor to ensure that children who need help always have someone to turn to at school. In addition all children who have been abused must have access to specialist therapeutic services to help them overcome their experiences. It is estimated that 90 per cent of children who have been sexually abused do not get any counselling or therapeutic support.
>
> (NSPCC 2007)

The need for a broad, universal system, as advocated by the NSPCC with in-schools therapists as a norm, and for the provision of clear referral is starkly illustrated by the criticisms identified by the Children's Society's *'Good Childhood' Enquiry*. The Report stated:

> Families also tell us that time and again when they were looking for advice, support and assistance they were turned away until the challenges overwhelmed them to the point of placing their children at risk. In the vast majority of cases, such risks are avoidable if supportive services are provided much earlier when they are requested.
>
> (2009: 29)

As part of the consultation a number of organizations and groups of children were included. The Department of Health asked the National Children's Bureau to consult with children and young people about what they thought of health and care services, what they thought was important to young children and what improvements could be made. The children said:

> They shouldn't make assumptions about what you want.
> They should let you choose who you want to be told about your loss/what kind of extra support you want.
> It helps if teachers are nice to you and try to show they understand.
> They should try to understand what you're going through and not be so tough about homework and things – it doesn't help.
>
> (DoH 2003: 29)

The need for universal access to therapy for children when needed was echoed by this report, commissioned by the UK Government and drawing on research with the users of child and adolescent mental health services (DoH 2003). It reported on key themes concerning accessible services, a first point of contact with someone who is well informed about the range of services for initial advice and referral, location within school buildings or in a situation that is both easy to get to and well publicized. The research noted from feedback from young people that 'contact with statutory settings can be experienced as stigmatizing and off putting' (2003: 5) and it recommended 'a holistic assessment and provision of services: multiple and different problem areas e.g. practical areas such as housing, schooling, alongside mental health issues' (2003: 5). It is within this set of drivers for change, foregrounding the necessity of accessible, appropriately designed, child-centred provision, that the need for dramatherapy can be placed.

The role of dramatherapy: two threes

The space for therapeutic support within schools is clearly an urgent and much needed priority. There are examples of practice in schools within the arts therapies and, specifically, dramatherapy (Case and Dalley 2008; Cefia and Cooper 2009; Jones 2010). Policy developments in related areas concerning children, interagency work and education and health all have the potential to impact favourably on dramatherapy provision. These range from dramatherapy services that are based outside schools but that children can access through school referral, services that work within schools to whole school approaches such as the social and emotional aspects of learning programme (SEAL), which can connect to dramatherapy in their form and delivery (National Advisory Council 2010).

Three main forms of dramatherapy in schools

Dramatherapy has become part of school life in the UK in three main forms. The forms are distinct from drama education:

> The arts therapist is distinct from an arts teacher . . . enabling the (child) to enter into the therapeutic opportunities and language of an arts therapy session. The main role of the therapist is not to teach, but to see how the client relates to the space and process, and to try to enable the maximum opportunities for arts therapy to occur.
>
> (Jones 2005: 204)

The first form is as a therapy offered to children who are in need of specific psychological intervention in relation to life events or issues. This route to dramatherapy is accessed by children who are dealing with issues in their lives such as bereavement or depression, or by children who may be communicating their response to complex emotional or social situations through behavioural difficulties. Carr and Ramsden summarize this area of work as follows:

> Dramatherapists in schools work with young people with a wide variety of needs, ranging from young children with a range of emotional and behavioural needs, to teenage girls who are self harming and adolescent boys who may have experienced violence in war-torn home countries.
>
> (2008: 167)

The second tends to involve children who come to dramatherapy to make use of the ways in which aspects of drama can enable therapeutic support for developmental assistance, or support in areas of growth and communication due to learning disability or physical impairment. The following describes interdisciplinary work between a teacher, dramatherapist and speech therapist with children with severe learning disabilities:

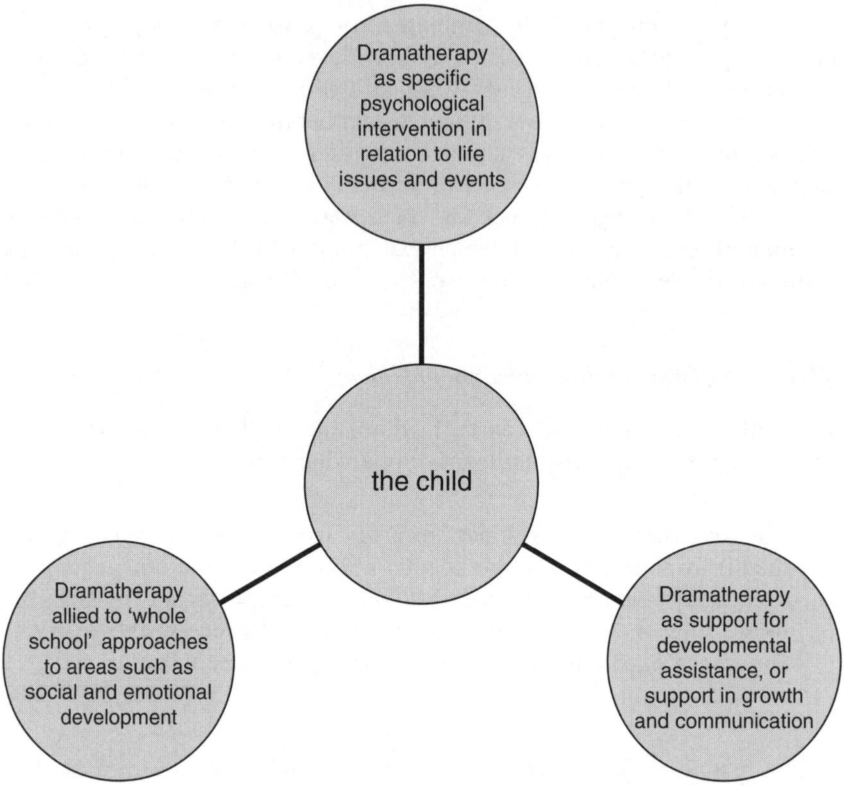

Figure 2.1 Dramatherapy: three main forms in schools

> Opportunities arose for role play, mime, expression of own identity and how each individual viewed himself, teamwork and story generation. . . . The children were able to practice functional language skills and creative skills in a non-threatening and stimulating situation, away from the constraints of a set agenda . . . They were also able to express feelings and fears verbally and non verbally in a safe and confident environment. The Speech and Language Therapist observed the children communicating in a novel environment, worked with them in a group situation, took part in new activities which naturally lent themselves to the use of higher language skills, and learned from another skilled professional who had a different but complementary approach to working with children with severe learning disabilities.
>
> (Chatterton and Butler 1994: 83)

Both of these forms tend to engage with children individually, or in groups, who are brought together with the therapist because of identified, specific needs or issues. The third form is allied to what has become known as a 'whole school' approach to areas such as social and emotional development and it concerns the ways in which dramatherapy can inform, or be part of, practice in areas such as SEAL and circle time. Mosely has written about the synergy between dramatherapy and circle time involving a whole school in group work that supports all children with proactive listening strategies such as 'speaking objects'; role play and puppetry; offering 'daily positive support through lunchtime availability of group work' and creating 'an open forum where children can safely share their feelings and ideas' (Mosely 2008: 2).

Examples of effective practice exist in each of these areas. Some schools liaise with external agencies providing dramatherapy for children, but that are located outside of the immediate school building and organization. Vaughan describes such a route to Family Futures, an organization that offers child and family therapy using the arts therapies:

> Colette was 13 years old when she was referred to Family Futures for an assessment because of absconding and school refusal. The referral had been triggered by an incident when the police picked up Colette late one night in a local park with a group of older boys who were taking drugs. Colette was already known to social services and the education welfare officer.
>
> (Vaughan in Jones 2007: 89)

In other schools dramatherapy is offered to groups and individuals through referral by adults or through self referral. Some schools employ dramatherapists, other schools may offer therapy through teachers who are also trained as a dramatherapist.

Dramatherapy as provision in schools: three key issues

In each of these ways of working there are three key issues that relate to the areas raised earlier in this chapter.

Firstly, the development of arts therapies such as dramatherapy in schools can be seen from a historical point of view as a key element of the move towards interdisciplinarity and the school as a site of multi-agency working. Secondly, the offering of dramatherapy in, or through, schools represents a vision of education that is allied to those that are child-centred, which sees our society's relationship to children and their education as necessarily more complex than as a subject- and target-driven domain. It acknowledges children as having a right to experiences in schools that enable them to develop and emerge in ways that have dialogue with the complexities of their lives, and in ways that reductionist approaches to schooling and school life do not. The provision of dramatherapy is allied to the approaches outlined earlier that emphasize that the interests of the child are prioritized and that the therapy is not seen solely through the prism of adult frameworks and

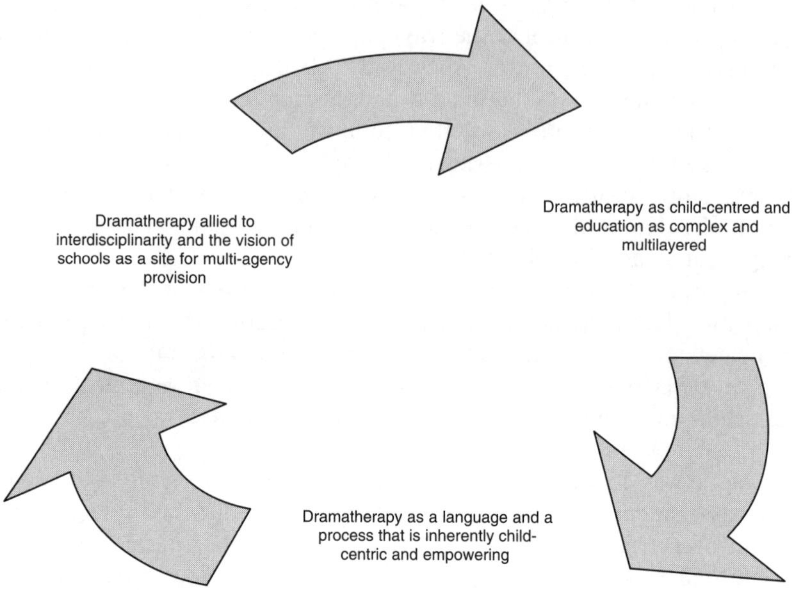

Figure 2.2 Dramatherapy as provision in schools: Three key issues

ideas. Thirdly, dramatherapy naturally lends itself to a child-centric approach that offers a child the opportunity to be an empowered, active agent in their own lives rather than a passive recipient of adult-delivered services. Dramatherapy enables the domain of the child to be valued and prioritized. Within therapy this can be seen to relate to the language and processes at work within the provision offered. If, as has been argued elsewhere, children turn to play and enactment to reflect and participate in their world, then play and enactment are natural forms for the child to inhabit and hence this mode of expression and communication prioritizes their concerns within their domain (Jones 2009b). Dramatherapy's language derives from play, the natural language for their assimilation of the world, their expression of their experiences and their ways of forming relationships with others. In this way it is both child-centric and empowering.

Developments such as the *National Services Framework* have this vision of dramatherapy's three ways of working and three key issues within its reach. So, for example, dramatic activity is cited in the Government summaries of effective case studies within the Department of Health's Case Study system for *the National Service Framework for Children, Young People and Maternity Services* (DoH and DfES 2006). Such work is linked to Standard 9 'The Mental Health and Psychological Well-being of Children and Young People'. The material focuses upon areas allied to those discussed in this chapter, such as whole school staff support and training to increase staff knowledge of mental health issues. The provision also includes what are called 'targeted interventions', which focus on groups of children who have known risk factors (individually or in their families) or on children at times of transition, for example from primary to secondary school (DoH and DfES 2006). Examples of these are given as a 'transition' group to reduce pupils' anxiety whilst helping with peer relationships, and a social skills group. Individual/family interventions are included and are described as usually 'involving Child and Adolescent Mental Health specialists for children who have already been identified as having specific difficulties' (DoH and DfES 2006). These are given as a drop-in clinic and individual work with children run by specialists. The usefulness of active methods and, specifically, drama are included within the provision through an after school club and drama workshops to increase social confidence. Another example given by the National Services Framework as a Case Example is the Place2Be – offering emotional and therapeutic support to children and parents in schools (DoH and DfES 2006).

Conclusion

The future of dramatherapy in schools, and in children's lives, is related to the ways in which the issues identified within this chapter are engaged with. These include how the culture-wide tensions within countries such as the UK develop: between education, therapy and childhood. Issues such as whether the call for the universal availability of therapy as a basic provision in schools is responded to rely on the interplay between complex factors. The availability of funding for dramatherapy reflects, for example, cultural attitudes to what a school is for and to political trends in policy. It also can reflect the innovative pressures coming from children and adults alike, who are identifying the potentials and the necessity of therapeutic provision in schools.

This chapter has shown the ways in which a dynamic shift is in progress, whereby schools and children may be seen differently: traditional processes of division and separation of education, health and play are challenged. Dramatherapy is a natural and necessary inhabitant of the changed school space envisioned by these shifts in attitude and ideas.

References

Archard, D. and Macleod, C. (2002) *The Moral and Political Status of Children*. Oxford: Oxford University Press.

Bottery, M. (1990) *The Morality of the School*. London: Cassell.

Carr, M. and Ramsden, E. (2008) 'An exploration of supervision in education', in P. Jones and D. Dokter (eds.), *Supervision of Dramatherapy*, 167–184. London: Routledge.

Case, C. and Dalley, T. (2008) *Art Therapy with Children*. London: Routledge.

Cefia, C. and Cooper, P. (eds.) (2009) *Promoting Emotional Education: Engaging*

Children and Young People with Social, Emotional and Behavioural Difficulties. London: Jessica Kingsley Press.

Chatterton, S. and Butler, S. (1994) 'The development of communication skills through drama', *Down Syndrome Research and Practice*, 2 (2), 83–84.

Children's Society (2009) *The Good Childhood enquiry: What children told us*. Available at: www.childrensociety.org.uk/resources/documents. Accessed 21 November 2009.

Cross, R. (2008) 'Provision for child health', in P. Jones, D. Moss, P. Tomlinson, and S. Welch (eds.), *Childhood: Services and Provision for Children*. Harlow: Pearson.

Department for Education and Skills (2003) *Every Child Matters*. London: Department for Education and Skills. London: The Stationery Office.

Department for Education and Skills (2004) *The Children Act*. London: The Stationery Office.

Department for Education and Skills (2007) *The Children's Plan*. London: The Stationery Office.

Department of Health (2003) *National Framework for Children, Young People and Maternity Services: Report from Consultation with Users of Child and Adolescent Mental Health Services*. London: The Stationery Office.

Department of Health (2005) *National Service Framework for Children, Young People and Maternity Services*. London: Department of Health.

Department of Health and Department for Education and Skills (2006) *Promoting the mental health and psychological well-being of children and young people: report on the Implementation of Standard 9 of the National Service Framework for Children, Young People and Maternity Services*. London: Department of Health. Available at: http://www.childrensnsfcasestudies.dh.gov.uk/children/nsfcasestudies.nsf. Accessed 21 November 2009.

Jones, P. (2005) *The Arts Therapies*. London: Routledge.

Jones, P. (2007) *Drama as Therapy*. London: Routledge.

Jones, P. (2009a) *Rethinking Childhood*. London: Continuum.

Jones, P. (2009b) 'Opening Play: research into play and dramatherapy', in A. Brock, S. Dodds, P. Jarvis, and Y. Olusoga (eds.), *Perspectives on Play: Learning for Life*. Harlow: Pearson.

Jones, P. (ed.) (2010) *Drama as Therapy 2*. London: Routledge.

Jones, P. and Welch, S. (2010) *Rethinking Children's Rights*. London: Continuum.

Laming, Lord (2003) *The Victoria Climbie Enquiry*. London: The Stationery Office.

Mosley, J. (2008) 'Setting up and running circles of support', *Social, Emotional and Behavioural Difficulties Association News*, 15, 1–4.

Moss, P. (2003) 'Re-forming the Education and Care Workforce in England, Scotland and Sweden', *UNESCO Policy Brief on Early Childhood*, 13, 1–2.

National Advisory Council (2010) *One Year On: the First Report from the National Advisory Council for Children's Mental Health and Psychological Wellbeing*. Available at http://nationaladvisorycouncilcmh.independent.gov.uk. Accessed 10 November 2010.

National Society for the Prevention of Cruelty to Children (2007) *NSPCC Welcomes the Children's Plan*. Available at http://www.nspcc.org.uk/whatwedo/mediacentre/pressreleases/2007_11_december. Accessed 21 January 2009.

Prout, A. (2000) 'Children's participation: control and self-realisation in British late modernity', *Children and Society*, 14, 304–315.

Rogers, W. (2004) 'Promoting better childhoods: constructions of child concern', in M. Kehily (ed.), *An Introduction to Childhood Studies*. Maidenhead: Open University Press.

Tomlinson, P. (2008) 'The politics of childhood', in P. Jones, D. Moss, P. Tomlinson, and S. Welch (eds.), *Childhood: Services and Provision for Children*. Harlow: Pearson.

Wahidin, A. and Moss, D. (2004) 'Women: Doing time and making time – reclaiming time', *International Journal of Sociology and Social Policy*, 24 (6), 76–111.

Welch, S. (2008) 'Education: service or system?' in P. Jones, D. Moss, P. Tomlinson, and S. Welch (eds.), *Childhood: Services and Provision for Children*. Harlow: Pearson.

3 Dramatherapy and drama teaching in school – a new perspective: towards a working relationship

Clive Holmwood and Carla Stavrou

Introduction

Traditionally dramatherapists and drama teachers in mainstream secondary schools have been seen to have very different roles. Dramatherapy within schools has most often been about an external qualified therapist going in to undertake an intervention for a child, or group of children, with an identified area of special need. This work often, but not always, takes place within the context of a specialist school for children who have learning, emotional or behavioural difficulties. Commonly the therapist provides a reflective therapeutic space in which group members have time and permission to think about thoughts, feelings and emotions within the context of the relationship, using drama with specific boundaries. Drama teachers have a more traditional educative role using drama didactically, which may be creative, developmental or curriculum-based – dependent on their individual and school emphasis – and as an aid to learning within a wider context. For this reason dramatherapists and drama teachers have sometimes been uneasy bedfellows.

This chapter brings together the perspectives, experience and research of a dramatherapist (Clive Holmwood) and an educational psychologist (Dr Carla Stavrou) to explore the potential for dialogue between drama teachers and dramatherapists in an educational context, and to consider how discussion between them may aid both professions and the students they work with.

Drama teaching and dramatherapy

There is a long history of debate about the purpose of drama as it features in education, central to which is the dichotomy between a traditional teacher-centred production/performance-driven approach and a student-centred process. In other words, whether drama should be about developing children as 'professional' actors, or if the educational value of drama is in the imaginary nature of the experience itself (Weltsek-Medina 2008). The latter approach has become known variously as Process Drama,

Applied Theatre and Drama in Education. Two leading practitioners and theorists of this approach are Dorothy Heathcote and Gavin Bolton, who emphasized how drama enables children to 'put themselves into another person's shoes', thus facilitating the development of insight and understanding (Heathcote 1995), and in this way becomes a medium through which any life experience may be explored (Bolton 1979). Over the past 40 years much has been written about how process drama can help children to safely explore identities, understand others' perspectives, reflect, make decisions and rehearse behaviours (Neelands 2004; Holland 2009). Descriptions such as these would appear to indicate that process drama, rather than drama aimed at teaching technical skills and culminating in a performance, is most relevant to this chapter. However, modern writers such as Gallagher state that students in dramatic performances in the classroom 'made explicit the dialogical relationship between the material subject (and her/his histories) and the imagined one' (2007: 8). This suggests that students are making connections between personal history within their community, and the imagined created drama. Thus drama has the potential to be a personal journey for each individual, allowing them to connect with their own stories and narratives. This, it could be argued, is closer to a more therapeutic or dramatherapy approach. Support for this can be found in the results of a study undertaken in a number of secondary schools by Stavrou (2010). Interviews with Heads of Drama working in secondary schools in Hertfordshire indicated that some pupils use the devised work element of their GCSE Drama course therapeutically by bringing material from their own lives to be worked through and rehearsed. One participating drama teacher related how 'I had a couple of boys in GCSE this year struggling with depression but able to bring some of that to the drama sometimes' (Stavrou 2010: 99), whilst another, describing a piece of work about bullying, reported that 'some of those students who have joined that group are students who actually feel threatened and bullied' (2010: 100).

Heathcote provides a drama teacher's perspective on the 'process versus product' dichotomy of drama in the classroom, suggesting that drama teachers operate in a 'vulnerable state' (Johnson and O'Neil 1989: 28). She points out that they struggle to communicate to colleagues issues between the process of how students learn and the actual results that can be assessed. Some drama teachers may consider that the process of drama is of greater importance, whereas others may feel the product, which may show more clearly specific skills that have been learnt, is more important (see Bolton 1988; O'Toole 1992). There is a deeper process at work, Heathcote states: 'many head teachers still think of it [drama] as watered down theatricals . . . because they themselves have only seen theatricals, or done theatricals in their own time in school' (Johnson and O'Neil 1989: 31).

Heathcote feels that a drama teacher 'must not only understand how to obtain progression in the work but also the difference between linear development in playmaking, the flow of the story line, the unfolding of events in true dramatic form, and the volume development of the work so that the events are personally meaningful to the children' (Johnson and O'Neil 1989: 31). The process of learning in drama is therefore not only about following a logical sequence with a dramatic story, and its pace and meter, character and plot, but about pulling out from this 'meaningful' elements of the story for the students in dramatic context. Interestingly, a number of the participants in Stavrou's research expressed the view that drama's non-statutory status allowed them the autonomy and flexibility to do just this. They reported planning and targeting schemes of work to meet the needs of a class, responding to requests to create tailored interventions within their lessons, and creating opportunities for pupils to take a lead in their own learning.

In the absence of a statutory subject framework for teaching Drama, individual secondary schools vary in the way they approach the subject. For example, they may teach drama as a part of English (Neelands 2004). Peter Slade, a pioneer in drama education, who first coined the phrase dramatherapy, suggests that from the beginning children should take note of the 'short sharp sounds which are equivalent of consonants and the long rich sounds which are equivalent of vowels' (1995: 50). He states children should learn to 'enjoy' language through English (1995: 106). One of Jones' nine core dramatherapy processes describes the dramatic body: the importance of the relationship between the body and the individual; the regulation of the body by society; and the way in which the body expresses itself and communicates (Jones 1996: 151). The construction of this within a social context is core work within dramatherapy. It could be argued that drama within English is not dissimilar to Jones's description of the dramatic body, finding its own way of connecting and communicating with the world outside. Language is a natural extension of the body.

Historically Slade's perception of drama teaching differed from that of more formal approaches, which relied on 'often received, standard or BBC speech' (Bolton 1988: 25). From the very beginning there was conflict between play and improvisational approaches, and formal speech and language. Neelands (2004) asserts that in schools where drama is used as a personal and social education, there is an emphasis on boosting social skills and personal relationships. This view is borne out by many of the accounts gathered by Stavrou in her research (2010). One Head of Drama described their subject as being 'about teaching social skills . . . teaching children how to listen to each other, how to respect each other, how to accept each other's differences and different strengths' (2010: 90). According to Neelands, drama used in this way in turn impacts on levels of self-esteem in what might be socially deprived areas. Drama in this kind of school would closely reflect the ethos of the school and community.

The subject of drama and the teaching of it within schools is pulled in a range of different directions. This has been influenced by government strategy and the subsequent development of the education system over recent decades, coupled with the influence of early drama pioneers who believed in the personal and social development of the individuals and groups through drama. Other writers suggest more structured approaches to drama, with it occupying a more central position within the curriculum as a contribution to English and other subjects. Finally, some see drama being taught as a subject within its own right. How drama is delivered in schools will of course also be influenced by the training, experiences and beliefs of individual drama teachers.

Dramatherapy in school

Karkou advises that there are already historical links between the arts therapies and education. 'The contribution of child centred education, with its emphasis upon emotional and social development, has enabled the development of arts therapies in this country' (2010: 10). Arts therapies were seen as 'sensitive' forms of arts teaching – a belief which, despite the professional development of the arts therapies, continues to exist. Karkou is right in that there is a 'willingness' for the development of social and emotional work within education, which has been developed in the guise of Personal, Social and Health Education and a raft of other legislation over recent years.

The idea of finding individual meaning from drama is very much core to dramatherapy. Jones states: 'The drama does not serve the therapy. The drama process contains the therapy' (1996: 4). The role of the drama-therapist is to assist individuals to make personal psychological connections to dramatic material, often from a psychodynamic perspective at an individual emotional level, whereas the drama teacher's role is to assist in the student's personal learning through drama.

The concept of process versus product may not be as clear in drama-therapy as it is in the classroom. Dramatherapists would generally be more interested in the process and less interested in creating a finished piece. This may be tempered by the training and background of the dramatherapist. A dramatherapist trained from a theatre background may be more interested in the dramatic technique and how this can be used to create meaning, whereas the dramatherapist from a psychological background may be more interested in the insight that can be made using the dramatic material.

Quibell (Karkou 2010) suggests the idea of using dramatherapy within a 'whole school set up'. He cites Action Group Skills (AGS) (2010: 115) as a way of using therapeutic work to aid 'whole school culture'. His research included children who showed concerning behaviour within the classroom who took part in an 11-week dramatherapy intervention. Quibell used a random control trial with half of the selected children taking part in dramatherapy intervention using the work of Jennings, Heathcote, Moreno and Emunah. The other half took part in small curriculum study groups.[1] His conclusions through observation and statistical analysis of questionnaire data from teachers, parents and pupils concluded that the dramatherapy approach was effective in the short *and* longer term (more than one year).

In a Canadian dramatherapy research project (Rousseau et al. 2007) a 9-week study was devised to look at the effectiveness of preventing emotional and behavioural problems and to enhance performance amongst immigrants and refugees. The Strength and Difficulties Questionnaire (SDQ) (Goodman 2001) was used to assess each student's level of emotional and behavioural distress before and after the dramatherapy intervention. Statistical analysis of the SDQs concluded that the dramatherapy work did not impact directly on the emotional and behavioural difficulties but did impact on the overall perception of impairment of symptoms (Rousseau et al. 2007: 461).

The main emphasis in these studies is the impact of dramatherapy in helping young people manage themselves socially and emotionally in the wider school environment. Quibell reported a positive impact some 12 months post project. Rousseau's work acknowledges that only short-term impact was assessed.

A common thread – and the importance of dramatherapy de-roling

It is important to acknowledge here a common thread identified within the reports of a number of the participants in the research undertaken by Stavrou concerning the tension between the therapeutic properties of drama and the school setting. One interviewee said 'I don't know how easy it would be to do something therapeutic in a school; essentially you need a neutral space where that child doesn't feel an association with failure' (2010: 100). Another interviewee spoke about covering emotive material in a drama lesson, highlighting the practical constraints of the school timetable: 'you've got to have time to deal with that situation before they go on to another class' (2010: 100). Comments such as these highlight an important distinction between the dramatherapist and the drama teacher. The dramatherapist is trained in how to de-role the client so that in a school setting the child returns to the classroom feeling a sense of balance, ready for class after dramatherapy. Drama teachers on the other hand do not have this training and need to be very careful if they are working with emotive material with a pupil or group of pupils.

The drama teacher and the dramatherapist

If a useful dialogue is to develop between drama teachers and dramatherapists, we may also wonder what similarities and differences exist between them. Koltai (Schattner and Courtney 1981) states a good teacher will possess some therapeutic skills just as a good therapist has to be able to teach. However, we would caution this view; being therapeutic does not make you a therapist, and not all therapists would agree they need to be able to teach. Courtney suggests 'intuition has particular significance because drama and creative arts educators claim a predominance of intuition in their thinking' (1989: 198). And they 'claim that it is their practical knowledge of drama and the arts that provides them with their unique perspective' (1989: 199). A striking regularity identified by Stavrou during thematic analysis of her interview data concerned the passion many drama teachers expressed for their subject, their previous experiences of working with young people with special educational needs, and a common willingness to address pupils' personal issues as they arose in school. The majority of interviewees cited personal attributes that helped to do this, which can be summarized as either life-experience or their own high level of social and emotional skills. Furthermore, it emerged in the course of the data collection that one of the ten participating teachers was considering re-training as a dramatherapist, and another was married to a practising dramatherapist.

However, teacher training and dramatherapy training are different in approach and intention. Dramatherapy students are expected to develop an understanding of self through personal therapy, which is an essential part of their training. Drama teachers are not. Dramatherapists are equipped to allow the client to work with their internal emotional and psychological world. The teacher will use a curriculum to teach students to develop personal, social and most importantly educational skills.

Dramatherapists come from a wide range of backgrounds and are expected to have either a first degree in a relevant subject or prove they have had significant experience in a related field before training. Once qualified, it is a legal requirement that they be registered with the Health Professions Council. A dramatherapist might have a background in drama, theatre, counselling, health or psychology. Therefore their background begins to shape them as individuals before, during and after training. Trainings will have a different emphasis dependent upon course and tutor. Approaches in the UK are defined as: theatre model (Holmwood's own training, though now unavailable, at Hertfordshire University), ritual theatre model, sesame approach, and integrated and eclectic approaches.[2] In the same way that the culture of the drama teacher within schools is shaped by a complex web of internal and external influences, from process or product and the social and political positioning of the school in its community, so too is the culture of dramatherapy. This has a huge impact upon the way a therapist or teacher may work or respond.

Edges in drama and dramatherapy

We have suggested that there are a range of differing approaches to drama in schools that have potential connections to dramatherapy. It has also been suggested that the training of the drama teacher and the drama-therapist is complex and is relational to the individual teacher or therapist's background and philosophical approach. There is a merging of philosophy and practice for teacher and therapist from their differing perspectives, which is worthy of further debate. We are not saying that drama teachers and dramatherapists are the same – but we do suggest an exploration of the space between and around each profession would be of benefit to all.[3]

Disabled performance artist Alicia Grace (2009), in an article entitled 'Dancing with latitude – a dramaturgy from limbo', discusses movement and dance and the friction created by artists operating on 'edges'. She states:

> According to the laws of permaculture, edges in the landscape are important because they are interfaces between two different types of environment or habitat. They share characteristics of both adjacent areas but have a unique character of their own. Edge eco-systems are known for their diversity and intense activity, they are also characterised as places of accumulation.
>
> (2009: 28)

The worlds of drama teaching and dramatherapy appear to have a potentially mutual impact for each other when their 'edges' meet and are acknowledged. A profession well-placed to occupy or bridge the gap between these edges might be educational psychology. Educational psychologists use their knowledge of psychological and therapeutic approaches to improve outcomes for all children. Much of this work is done in and with schools, and is focused on children and young people who are experiencing barriers to enjoying, achieving and developing during their time in education. Thus, educational psychologists have some knowledge of therapeutic approaches and considerations, and experience of using interventions to support young people with identified additional needs. At the same time they also offer knowledge and experience of the school and its context. We suggest that this combination means that they are in an excellent position for supporting a dialogue between dramatherapists and drama teachers, with the aim of enriching both professions and enhancing their effectiveness.

Conclusion

There is evidence to suggest that social and emotional learning interventions yield multiple benefits relating to each of the five outcomes of Every Child Matters (Department for Education and Skills 2003). It is imperative for educational psychologists and other professionals to support schools to develop and implement interventions that are effective in promoting social and emotional development. It is particularly important to identify interventions that use resources and expertise already located in schools. We feel that the findings of Stavrou's research provide evidence that drama's non-statutory status allows teachers the autonomy and flexibility to use their subject to address issues as they arise within their classes, or to tailor schemes of work to target identified areas of need. Whilst there is evidence that some teachers experience their subject as enabling therapeutic change for some pupils, many acknowledged the tensions and limitations associated with the therapeutic properties of drama and the school setting. Finally, we propose that beyond providing an evidence base for using drama to develop social skills and empathy in secondary school pupils, the findings of this study raise awareness about the knowledge, experience, skills and techniques located within school drama departments, which could contribute to development and implementation of interventions for improving outcomes for pupils.

Despite differences in the nature, training and intention of the drama teacher and dramatherapist, and the political and social contexts around them, they both share one thing in common – the art form, drama. Just as each profession has its own boundary or 'edge' as Grace suggests, one environment can have an impact on the other. What needs to be developed further is the opportunity in schools to allow each profession not only to understand their own boundary and that of the other, but also to acknowledge the space between them, and what this is. As Grace writes, 'edge ecosystems are not only places of "intense activity" but also of "accumulation"'.

Notes

1 Quibell notes that random control groups using therapeutic group work are rare.
2 As listed in the British Association of Dramatherapists' website training table. Available at http://www.badth.org.uk/training/table.html, Accessed 23 January 2011.
3 This is the site of Clive Holmwood's doctoral research.

References

Bolton, G. (1979) *Towards a Theory of Drama in Education*. London: Longman.

Bolton, G. (1988) *Drama as Education – An Argument for Placing Drama at the Centre of the Curriculum*, second edition. London: Longman.

Courtney, R. (1989) *Play Drama and Thought: the Intellectual background to Dramatic Education* – fourth edition revised. Toronto: Simon & Piere.

Department for Education and Skills (2003) *Every Child Matters*. London: HMSO.

Gallagher, K. (2007) *The Theatre of Urban – Youth and Schooling in Dangerous Times*. Toronto: University of Toronto Press.

Goodman, R. (2001) 'Psychometric properties of the Strengths and Difficulties Questionnaire (SDQ)'. *Journal of the American Academy of Child and Adolescent Psychiatry*, 40, 1337–1345.

Grace, A. (2009) 'Dancing with lassitude: A dramaturgy from limbo'. *Research in Drama Education: The Journal of Applied Theatre and Performance*, 14, 15–29.

Heathcote, D. (1995) *Drama for Learning*. London: Heinemann.

Holland, C. (2009) 'Reading and acting in the world: Conversations about empathy'. *Research in Drama Education: The Journal of Applied Theatre and Performance*, 14, 529–544.

Johnson, L. and O'Neil, C. (ed.) (1989) *Dorothy Heathcote – Collected Writings on Education and Drama*. London: Hutchinson.

Jones, P. (1996) *Drama as Therapy Theatre as Living*. London: Routledge.

Karkou, V. (ed.) (2010) *Arts Therapies in Schools. Research and Practice*. London: Jessica Kingsley.

Neelands, J. (2004) *Beginning Drama*, second edition. London: David Fulton.

O'Toole, J. (1992) *The Process of Drama: Negotiating Art & Meaning*. London: Routledge.

Rousseau, C., Benoit, M., Gauthier, M.F., Lacroix, L., Alain, N., Viger Rojas, M., Moran, A., and Bourassa, D. (2007) 'Classroom drama therapy program for immigrant and refugee adolescents: A pilot study'. *Clinical Child Psychology and Psychiatry*, 12, 451–465.

Schattner, G. and Courtney, R. (1981) *Drama in Therapy. Vols. 1 & 2*. New York: Drama Book Specialist.

Slade, P. (1995) *Child Drama*. London: Jessica Kingsley.

Stavrou, C. (2010) *An Investigation into How Drama is Used to Develop Young People's Empathy and Social Skills in Secondary Schools*. Unpublished doctoral thesis, University of East London (UEL).

Weltsek-Medina, G.J. (2008) 'Process Drama in Education: General Considerations', in Blatner, A. (ed.), *Interactive and Improvisational Drama: Varieties of Applied Drama and Performance*. Bloomington: I Universe Inc.

4 Supporting children in primary school through dramatherapy and the creative therapies

Brenda Meldrum

Introduction

What do children need most of all? They need love. If a child is loved, she thinks she is lovable, she can love herself and she can love other people. If a child has no-one to love him and cannot remember anyone who has loved him, then he is in mental turmoil and is deeply, deeply unhappy. Our emotions are reflected in our behaviour; in school the children who are unhappy and angry or depressed at the way they are treated will express their feelings directly in their relationships with teachers, support staff and other children. We all desire and need to make relationships with others, and in schools, the impact of early relationships, secure and insecure, are played out in the classroom and in the playground.

In this chapter I shall briefly give the case for early intervention and then look at the current literature that addresses the experiences of children and young people in school. The basis of my approach as a dramatherapist is through the lens of John Bowlby's theory of Attachment and Loss (Bowlby 1988). I shall look at the concerns for the mental health of our school children and how we make positive relationships with them, and I shall examine the skills that we need as dramatherapists and arts therapists when working with young people. Later in this book, I present a model of the ways in which we can support children and staff in primary school, and the huge role that dramatherapists, art therapists and play therapists can play in supporting the emotional development of children.

The case for early intervention

The perception of many of us who work in schools giving emotional support to children is that the number of children whose behaviour is causing concern to staff is increasing. Reception teachers in the schools where I work, and whose staff I train, report that children often have very poor social, communication and language skills and seem to have difficulty in managing their emotions.

The Department for Children, Schools and Families (2010) said there is evidence that when children and young people's emerging difficulties are not spotted and addressed early on they become entrenched and may spiral and multiply, causing significant long-term damage for them and for others around them. Not only does this cause unhappiness but it can create big financial costs for a wide range of public services far into the future. Early intervention means intervening as soon as possible to tackle problems that have already emerged for children and young people and that are getting in the way of their learning. Schools are often the places where emerging difficulties are first spotted, or where children and young people or their families will themselves seek help. Schools are also the most appropriate setting within which the extra help children need can be delivered. When the high costs of 'non-intervention' are compared with the significantly lower costs of intervening early, it becomes clear that early intervention is the better approach.

Working one to one or in small groups, dramatherapists and other arts and play therapists give emotional support to children and young people in schools. I have listened to the argument that working only with the child one to one does not address the social, family and environmental issues that is the context and may be the cause of her emotional needs, but I believe in the power of active listening, of empathy and compassion, of communication through play and drama and of making a relationship to help the young person find strategies and the resilience to cope with their often difficult lives. Teachers and staff report to me that the young people's emotional arousal is lower after coming to sessions; this emphasizes the importance of the relationship between the therapist and the child where the adult, in her 'parent-like role' acts as container of the child's emotional reactions.

Current literature on the experiences of children

The Demos Report (2010) for Barnardos

In June 2010, the think tank Demos, in association with Barnardos, wrote a report called *In Loco Parentis* (Hannon et al. 2010) in which it was stated that 55 children in England per every 10,000 are looked after by the local authority. Martin Narey, the Chief Executive of Barnardos at the time, as a result of the Demos report called for:

- early intervention
- fewer family placements and long stays in care
- age of leaving care to be raised from 16 to 18 years.

Children in care attend school and their attachment difficulties, their unhappiness and their inability to find meaning in what is happening to them are inevitably expressed in their behaviour and in their perceptions of themselves. Demos reports that, in 2009, 10.7% of looked-after children had three or more placement moves in a year, 67% were in a long-term placement (defined as more than 2.5 years) and many young people experienced up to 10 placement moves. The school I work in relies on its arts therapists, and students on placement, to work one to one and in small groups with looked-after children.

The Landmark Report for the Children's Society (2009)

One of the most interesting commentaries on the way we in the United Kingdom treat our children is the Landmark Report for the Children's Society *A Good Childhood: Searching for Values in a Competitive Age* (Layard and Dunn 2009). Despite the almost hysterical media opposition to its thesis that in order to bring up children so that they are not only happy but also are able to fulfil their potential, *adults* have to change, the intelligent reader recognizes that it is a down-to-earth and commonsense application of research to practice. This report presents evidence that suggests that more young people are anxious and troubled; that more young people have behavioural problems and that these problems are connected with the changing world in which children are growing up. Some of the changes that are common are:

- Family break up.
- Mothers working [sic].
- Exposure to new media including the Internet.
- Commercial and lifestyle advertising and influence.
- Pressure of school examinations.
- Increasing relative poverty.

The authors agree that some of the widespread unease about the commercial pressures exerted on children, the violence they are exposed to on film, DVD and on the internet, the stresses at school and the threats to their safety from predatory adults is exaggerated and 'reflects unwarranted angst about the greater freedom that children now enjoy' (p. 1). There is, however, a genuine fear that children's lives are more difficult than they ought to be. They quote a UNICEF (2007) report on the life of children in 21 of the world's richest countries; in the overall ranking Britain was *bottom* and the United States next to bottom. It is worth looking more closely at the findings in this report as they apply to Britain because it will give us a background to some of the distress that children express in schools.

The UNICEF Innocenti Research Report (2007): Child Poverty in Perspective: an overview of child well-being in rich countries

The UNICEF report provides a comprehensive assessment of the lives and well-being of children and young people in 21 nations of the industrialized world. The report measures and compares overall child well-being across six dimensions: material well-being, health and safety, education, peer and family relationships, behaviours and risks, and young people's subjective perceptions of their own well-being. Of the 21 nations assessed, the United Kingdom is at the bottom of the ranking for child well-being. Furthermore, the UK ranks in the bottom third on five of the six dimensions reviewed:

- Material well-being, in terms of relative poverty and deprivation.
- Educational well-being, in terms of school achievement at age 15.
- Percentage of young people remaining in education and the transition to employment.
- Family and peer relationships, defined as the quality of children's relationships with their parents and peers.
- Behaviour and risk-taking in terms of health and risk behaviours and experience of violence.
- The last dimension, where the UK ranked 21st of all the nations, was the dimension assessing the children's own perception of their well-being in terms of their own health, their experience of school life and their personal well-being. The report makes alarming reading for those of us who are working with children and young people in the UK.

Among other findings in this report, the following are of particular interest:

- Nine northern European countries have brought relative child poverty rates below 5%. However, in three Anglophone countries (the UK, the US and Ireland), relative child poverty remains above 15%.
- While overall 80% of children live with both parents (more than 90% in Greece and Italy), less than 70% of children live with both parents in the UK.

UNICEF says the true measure of a nation's standing is:

> how well it attends to its children – their health and safety, their material security, their education and socialisation and their sense of being loved, valued, and included in the families and societies into which they are born.
>
> (2007: 1; Report Card 7)

It would seem we have a problem in Britain. What is the cause? According to the Good Childhood report, the common theme is *excessive individualism*. They argue that the pursuit of personal success relative to others cannot create a happy society, since one person's success involves another's failure and that in Britain the balance between individual freedom and responsibility for others has tilted too far towards the individual pursuit of private interest and success. They assert that it is excessive individualism that is causing high family break-up, teenage unkindness, unprincipled advertising, too much competition in education and our acceptance of income inequality, all of which affect our nation's children directly. The major theme of their report is that we need to change into a 'society based upon the law of love'.

The Good Childhood Inquiry recommends that parents should:

- Make a long-term commitment to each other.
- Be fully informed about what is involved before their child is born.
- Love their children and each other and establish boundaries for children.
- Help children develop spiritual qualities.

While they recognize that the first and key role of the school is to develop the powers of the mind, the authors stress that the second key role – and in their view of equal importance – is to train the habits of the heart, and to look after the emotional needs of young people. The research indicates that there is no conflict between the objectives of harmonious living and academic excellence; indeed, 'When inner calm is enhanced, better studying results' (p. 106). However, disruption in the classroom is one of the main impediments to learning and for most teachers the main issue is repeated low-level disruption and impoliteness, rather than knives or guns.

What can be done? The solution they propose is two-fold: first, the schools must act as values-based communities promoting mutual respect between all members within the school system and involving parents closely. Secondly, and equally important, schools should help individual pupils manage their emotions. A school should judge how successful it is in educating a pupil by her intellectual progress *and* her emotional development.

Children's emotional well-being and mental health in schools

How do we define emotional well-being? Tina Bruce (2005) suggests that a child's emotional well-being is dependent on being in a relationship with a caring and loving adult who both communicates with the child, and encourages communication with the adult. Brazelton and Greenspan, two eminent paediatricians and psychologists, say that 'Mental health involves family and school as well as other settings where the child is engaged in daily experiences' (2000: 143) and they suggest that most problems are associated with a lack of developmentally appropriate experiences in one form or another. They state that children who have problems with making relationships often have difficulty in reading social cues and signals. Some children have extreme emotional reactions, which means that they often have not mastered the ability to regulate their emotions. This is not their fault; it is always the adult's responsibility to help children manage their emotions and if they don't have this experience at home, then we have to try in school to be models of adults who can manage our own feelings and not allow them to spill over. Furthermore, these authors stress the importance of ongoing secure, empathic and nurturing relationships, which help children learn to be intimate and communicate their feelings and reflect upon their own wishes. Such relationships teach children which behaviours are appropriate and which are not. From birth children learn from their parents' facial expressions, tone of voice, gestures and then words which behaviours lead to approval or disapproval.

Layard and Dunn (2009) stress that children with mental health difficulties are often seriously troubled or disturbed, yet only a quarter of those affected are getting any kind of specialist help. The time to help children is early on, when their difficulties are less entrenched and when they are responsive to good interventions. This is where early intervention in primary schools can really assist the emotional well-being of children. These authors reviewed research on the key factors that directly affect mental health and I summarize their findings. Poorer children are more likely than others to have mental health difficulties, not because of lack of income itself, but because of other related difficulties, including:

- Living apart from the father, which increased the risk of difficulties by 40%.
- Family conflict.
- Poor mental health of a parent.
- Living in rented housing and
- More than two adverse life events.

> The strength of the family effect is particularly striking. In nearly every survey the proportion of children with behavioural difficulties is at least 50 per cent higher in families with single parents or step-parents than in families where both parents are still together.
>
> (2009: 117)

The papers I have quoted make it clear that schools in Britain are coping with children whose emotional well-being is being compromised by familial, cultural, societal and systemic factors that are causing them real unhappiness and distress. Because children have to go to school, it seems only rational to base therapeutic intervention – especially early intervention – in school settings.

John Bowlby's theory of attachment and loss

First and foremost is the bedrock thinking of Attachment Theory, defined originally by John Bowlby (1907–1990) and expanded by Mary Ainsworth (1913–1999) and increasingly important in today's world. John Bowlby was both a physician and a psychoanalyst who worked with, among others,

Anna Freud and Melanie Klein, before breaking away and founding his own theory based on observations and clinical practice with children, young people, their parents and above all their mothers. His clinical work was expanded through the research of Mary Ainsworth and her colleagues (1978) at Berkeley. There is a massive body of research around early and later attachment relationships and their importance to each human being's happiness and self-esteem. Conversely, speculation into the long-term effects of disruption in early relationships has become increasingly the subject of neurophysiological research, which has graphically demonstrated the effects of deprivation on the development of the human brain.

The core premises of John Bowlby's Attachment Theory (1988)

First, Bowlby said that human infants are pre-programmed to make attachments with the person who is caring for them. The human infant's behaviours develop into patterns that will promote the attachment relationship of adult and infant – behaviours like crying, clinging, eye contact and the developing behaviours of following, reaching and seeking proximity with the parent or carer. While any relationship is a two-way process, the responsibility for its development lies with the adult. The evolutionary purpose of these behaviours and this relationship is the survival of the infant through the protective behaviour of the adult. Thus, attachment relationships are part of our humanity. They cannot be avoided or downplayed, and they have to be recognized.

Attachment relationships and attachment behaviours are suffused with emotion 'irrespective of the age of the individual' (Bowlby 1988: 4). On the one hand, if the attachment relationship goes well and is secure, there is joy and security. If it is threatened, and when there is jealousy, anxiety and anger, or if it is broken – if the attachment is severed – there is grief, anger and depression. He suggests that the quality of early attachment relationships relate to our emotional functioning throughout our lives and within all our subsequent relationships. Thus, the self develops through the relationships we have with other people, which are in turn mediated by the communication we have with these people.

How do these core premises affect us as dramatherapists and arts therapists working within the school setting? How do we use Bowlby's insights to make relationships with young people and also with the teaching and support staff? What basic skills do we need to work with children and young people?

A professional who is applying Bowlby's attachment theory in her work sees her role as that of providing the *secure base*, the safety and the conditions in which the person can explore his or her internal representation of self and his attachment figures in such a way that they can be restructured as the client gains insights through his play and the experience of the relationship with the adult. First, we provide a secure base from which the person can explore emotions, thoughts and beliefs, which are sometimes difficult or impossible to talk about or even think or play about without support, encouragement, sympathy and guidance. Next, we assist the person in exploring the way in which they engage in relationships and what their expectations are for their own feelings and behaviour as well as how others will react to them.

The relationship between the dramatherapist and the child is the main way for the therapist to learn how the child operates with their primary attachment figure and in this relationship we need to be able to encourage the child to express these constructions and expectations. We allow the young people to experiment with the idea that the ways in which they think about themselves may be a product of the way they were parented, which is a difficult and emotional experience. However, because we work within the safety of the play and the drama, then we can contain these emotions and difficulties. We allow the young people to reassess their models of self and of others; then they may be able to understand that their constructions of self and their worlds is inaccurate and that there may be different ways of representing self and others.

As professionals we are responsible for the attunement and sensitivity of our responses to young people, and we can make appropriate and secure attachments with them, if we share a *nonverbal* focus on our emotional states and a *verbal* focus on the narratives of their mental lives.

Chris Taylor (2010) speaks of the need for adults working with young people to develop attunement with them and to show through our tone of voice, facial expression and body language that we see and appreciate the emotions the person is experiencing, acknowledging the emotions embedded in the person's story in simple non-judgemental statements, for example: 'I can see this is hard for you. . .' and we can gently reflect upon what the young person is telling us. Taylor reminds us that we block empathy when we try to stop the person from feeling pain because we don't want them to be distressed. But they are distressed and if we are empathic we try to understand how they feel – what it is like to be in their shoes – not to try and stop ourselves being upset because they are upset. If we show empathy and compassion for ourselves and for the young people we can build therapeutic relationships through mindfulness and attunement (Gilbert 2009).

Conclusion

Children come to school with different experiences; the way they are treated, especially in their early relationships within the family, helps or hinders their self-esteem and the way they feel about themselves. However, because young people are obliged to attend school, dramatherapists, embedded in a school's culture, can help find ways of supporting their emotional needs, which affect not only their learning but also their emotional well-being. This is how we can make a difference to their lives.

Acknowledgements

Demos, The Children's Society and UNICEF are kindly acknowledged.

References

Ainsworth, M., Blehar, M., Water, E., and Wall, S. (1978) *Patterns of Attachment: A Psychological Study of the Strange Situation*. Oxford: Lawrence Erlbaum.

Bowlby, J. (1988) *A Secure Base: Clinical Applications of Attachment Theory*. London: Routledge.

Brazelton, T.B. and Greenspan, S.I. (2000) *The Irreducible Needs of Children: What every child must have to grow, learn and flourish*. Cambridge, MA: Da Capo Press.

Bruce, T. (2005) *Learning Through Play*. London: Hodder Arnold.

Department for Children, Schools and Families (2010) *Early Intervention: Securing good outcomes for all children and young people*.

Gilbert, P. (2009) *The Compassionate Mind*. London: Constable & Robinson.

Hannon, C., Wood, C., and Bazalgette, L. (2010) *In Loco Parentis*. London: Demos.

Layard, R. and Dunn, J. (2009) *A Good Childhood: Searching for Values in a Competitive Age*. London: The Children's Society/Penguin Books.

Taylor, C. (2010) *A Practical Guide to Caring for Children and Teenagers with Attachment Difficulties*. London: Jessica Kingsley.

UNICEF (2007) *Child Poverty in Perspective. An Overview of Child Well-Being in Rich Countries*. Florence: UNICEF Innocenti Research Centre.

Part II

Case studies

5 Whizzing and whirring: dramatherapy and ADHD

Ann Dix

Working with a child with a diagnosis of attention deficit hyperactivity disorder (ADHD) can be a challenge to a dramatherapist. Current thinking is that these children need clear, boundaried work that helps to contain their behaviour and structure their thought processes. It is recognized that there needs to be different interventions to address different symptoms (Kapalka 2008), but children are usually offered a mixture of medication and Cognitive Behavioural Therapy (CBT). Some children may be offered group work to develop listening, concentration and impulse control; however, children with ADHD can also be creative and in this chapter I intend to use a case study to demonstrate that dramatherapy is an important intervention, enabling the creation of a symbolic and metaphoric reality that they can explore (Jones 2007).

ADHD refers to a range of problem behaviours associated with poor attention span and includes impulsiveness, restlessness and hyperactivity. It affects about 3% of the population, most of whom are boys, and recent research suggests that it may have a genetic element (Williams et al. 2010), although there is still widespread disagreement between professionals as to its causes (Biddulph 1997; Cooper and Bilton 1999). It also may co-exist alongside other emotional, behavioural or learning difficulties. ADHD requires a medical diagnosis, but because there is no single diagnostic test, different information needs to be collated from a variety of professional sources – these include the observations of teachers, learning mentors, therapists and psychologists – in order to rule out other reasons such as poor attachment patterns or autism. Often parents feel responsible for their child's behaviour, and whilst poor parenting and lack of attachment can produce similar symptoms to ADHD, most parents are not to blame and are at a loss to know how to cope. It is imperative that any work with the child also includes support for the family.

The behaviour patterns of ADHD usually emerge between the ages of three and five. Children are described as being 'always on the go', restless and unable to concentrate. In schools, this can lead to disruptive behaviour as children struggle to learn, often using distracting behaviours to mask their lack of understanding or their inability to concentrate. Children with

ADHD are frequently intelligent, and become frustrated as they fail to make the progress of which they are capable. For educators, these children can be infuriating to work with, as they may concentrate for long periods of time on something of interest to them but be unable to attend to concepts that do not originate in their own thought patterns. This can often set them up for failure in traditional classroom and therapy sessions that rely solely on verbal interactions (Chasen 2005: 154).

Children with ADHD like to remain in control 'and have difficulties accepting that rules must be arrived at by consensus' (Kapalka 2008: 163). They often have difficulty with peer friendships as they find it difficult to negotiate. These children are frequently seen as confrontational as they find it difficult to suppress the impulse to protest when they do not get their own way, leading them to be labelled as angry rather than reactive (Kapalka 2008: 166), yet they may also have low self esteem as a result of negative labelling (Cooper and Bilton 1999).

However, as we become more able to understand ADHD we are able to offer more effective support for the child. Increasingly, neurobiological research indicates that chemicals in the brain influence a whole range of behaviours; for example, dopamine plays a part in inhibiting impulsive behaviour and enhancing concentration (Cooper and Bilton 1999). Traditionally, the medical treatment for ADHD has been methylphenidate (e.g. Ritalin) or dexamfetamine (Dexedrine), which are class A amphetamine-like stimulants that reduce hyperactivity and impulsiveness in children and allow learning to take place; however, there are increasing concerns about the possible side effects, including weight loss, and possible damage to the cardiovascular and nervous systems.

So it would appear to be imperative that other forms of therapy, which create natural chemical changes in the brain and allow the child to develop new strategies for developing calmness and managing behaviour, are implemented. Bannister (2002; Bannister and Huntingdon 2003) believes that the brain has a 'plasticity' that allows for new synapses to be formed when the right brain is stimulated by emotional experiences. Research by Schore (2003) and Gerhardt (2004) have found that the orbitofrontal cortex, the part of the brain that controls impulses, is 'experience'-dependent (Gerhardt 2004: 38) and can only develop through relationships with others, thus allowing a mental space in which stress hormones can create new synapses in the higher cortex of the brain. Dramatherapy can stimulate the brain and help to develop new ways of behaving because it is action based and uses movement, symbol and metaphor rather than conventional talking, either through group work or interactions with the therapist.

Haen describes how dramatherapy allows themes to be actively embodied, thus 'creating novel associations in the brain and in forming new synaptic connections that can lead to altered perceptions, increased feelings of connection and an expanded sense of self' (2005: 223).

Dramatherapy can enable children to use symbolism and metaphor to express their feelings in a way that is safe and creative. It is particularly accessible to children whose verbal skills may not be well developed and whose self esteem may be low. Such children can access their creativity and use the play and storytelling to express themselves in new ways. Initially this may be non-verbal, which can develop into projection of character and themes onto creative materials that allow the child to externalize ADHD and begin to understand how it affects them.

Working as a dramatherapist with a child who has a diagnosis of ADHD can be very rewarding. The child who is frequently labelled as naughty can be helped to control their impulses and practice different ways of reacting to situations. They can be given an opportunity to be seen as a whole child, rather than primarily a child with ADHD. The therapist will require lots of energy and the ability to keep clear boundaries in order for the work to feel contained and they will need to create a therapeutic space that is calm and ordered to allow for the processing of ideas and creation of new thought patterns to emerge.

Dramatherapists often work individually with children where the personal nature of the metaphor can be maintained and explored (Langley 2006) and dramatherapy encourages the 'projection of an inner emotional trauma or problem into a dramatic representation' (Jones 2007: 138). Dramatic play is crucial to a child's development and the drama-developmental paradigm known as embodiment-projection-role (EPR; Jennings 1990, 1993, 1995) is a useful model when beginning a piece of work with a child. Mirroring the early developmental stages, it allows the child to move between the three areas as on a continuum (Jones 2007) and revisit any stage that may have been arrested. It also allows the child to have mastery over events and circumstances that might be beyond their control. 'Through dramatic play a child can reduce the world to a size where it is manageable and where the events of everyday reality can be played out in relative safety' (McFarlane 2005: 8).

In dramatherapy terms, sensory or embodiment play may involve movement, such as rolling or jumping, playdough and clay, or any physical action that involves the senses. Projective play may use any external object to tell stories, such as dolls, small figures, or may involve use of sand play and drawing. Role play will engage the child in storytelling 'as if' the child were someone else and allow the child to express their thoughts metaphorically. Role play often involves more than one person and therefore a dialogue develops between therapist and child, which stimulates the neuro pathways and encourages emotional intelligence (Goleman 1996) through what Chasen calls 'spectacle and ensemble', which challenges the children to manage their impulses and become more socially aware (Chasen 2005).

Group work may concentrate on social skills, impulse control and cooperation, and individual work involving the child and the therapist may seem very different. Sometimes the work can feel disjointed, as the child moves from place to place in the room, or from toy to toy. However, by staying with the child in the moment the dramatherapist may begin to see a pattern emerge.

The following case study describes a piece of dramatherapy with an individual child, Luke, who attended weekly sessions. It is a snapshot of work that lasted a year and concentrates on two aspects of the work. He attended sessions during the school day, and the school supported this by releasing him from lessons. During this time I liaised closely with Luke's class teacher and his family so that there was good communication between us and there were support systems in place. Luke's name and details have been changed.

Case study: Luke

Nine-year-old Luke had caused his parents and teachers concern for some time. When I first met him he was about to be assessed by child and adolescent mental health services (CAMHS) and he was diagnosed with ADHD halfway through my work with him. He attended a local primary school in the midst of a large housing estate, and was under-achieving. He was generally a popular boy with his peers, and although he was often in trouble for fighting, this was usually because he was trying to 'sort things out' for his friends. Luke had difficulties with impulsiveness, and found it almost impossible to sit still and not roam the classroom, fiddling with the computers or irritating his teacher and peers. When he was reprimanded for his behaviour, he often perceived it as a personal attack, which would make him very defensive. Luke's teachers found him argumentative and difficult to work with.

The referral was made to my team by Luke's school following discussions with his parents. A meeting was arranged with his mother in order to get a clearer picture of the difficulties Luke was experiencing, where it became apparent that Luke's family were very supportive of him and his school. His mother had attended a parenting course and was putting the suggestions into practice. She explained that Luke was a very affectionate child who enjoyed her company, but who had little concentration and who found it difficult to stay on task. She described how Luke would constantly ask her questions, seemingly forgetting the answers immediately. He was unable to sit and play board games, and became bored and restless when watching TV. She limited his use of the computer, where he enjoyed playing games, and tried to encourage him into physical activities to use up his energy. Even when Luke was asleep he appeared restless, and often talked in his sleep.

Luke agreed to come to weekly dramatherapy sessions, and appeared to enjoy them. The first few sessions were spent exploring the playroom and the toys. He seemed unable to engage with anything for very long and maintained a constant stream of excited chatter. I commented on what he was doing, but he seemed unable to listen.

Luke enjoyed playing with the playmobile people and rescue vehicles, creating elaborate chases and accidents which required helicopters and ambulances, and supplying a dizzying cacophony of sound effects. Sometimes it was difficult to follow the stories, as they moved around the room, and Luke would give me instructions about what I should be doing or saying. I tried to remain attuned, stopping him occasionally to clarify points or comment on something he was doing. Gradually, the stories became more coherent, and Luke was able to sustain concentration for longer. I asked him what his mother would say if she could see him playing so calmly and he replied that she would be amazed.

One day, on our way to the session, Luke spotted a large cardboard box in the corridor and asked if he could have it. We carried it into the play room, where he began a piece of work that carried on for several weeks. We had talked about how Luke's brain was a bit like a computer, thinking and processing information, but that sometimes it seemed to be whirring too fast, so that it felt as though he had little control over it. Luke liked this metaphor and we explored it further by thinking of all the different programmes running in his head, and how his thoughts and ideas became jumbled and tumbled over themselves. Luke thought about how he couldn't switch off his computer brain at night, therefore it continued whirring, even when he was asleep, so that he woke up feeling tired. The box was big enough for Luke to sit in, and he said that it was going to be his 'computer brain'.

Luke thought about how he tried to learn in class, and was able to describe some of his difficulties. He said that the noise of the light distracted him, so he began to tap his pencil to its rhythm until he broke the pencil point. Then, he needed to sharpen his pencil, but when he stood up, he knocked into the girl sitting next to him who pushed him back. He tried to tell the teacher, but she told him to sit down and stop being argumentative, and then he dropped his book on the floor, and so on; all day, every day. Luke became quite down-hearted, as he perceived that he couldn't get things right, even when he tried. His self esteem was very low and he was in danger of giving up altogether. He was also learning that his negative behaviours got him attention but that his positive attempts did not.

Luke began to examine the box. He cut a window in the side, to see the world through, and carefully divided the inside into different areas. He carefully constructed a shelf for pens and paper, as a learning area, and created a relaxation area, with a cushion for playing games and reading, as well as an area for keeping food and eating. He wrote different things on the walls of the box, which would make it a special and safe place to be inside. Luke also created a panel of dials, including one that said SLOW in big letters.

On the outside of the box he created a notice board for messages. This was for him to write reminders for himself, and for others to leave messages for him. He also added a cushion and drew flowers and a telephone. When it was completed, Luke was able to sit inside.

Luke created a symbolic representation of his ADHD, as a computer that sometimes went too fast for him to keep up with. He was able to incorporate some suggestions as to how he might begin to manage this, including a slow dial and a place to relax. As Jones states, 'Work involving symbol and metaphor in dramatherapy can help clients to engage in highly problematic material. They serve both to permit expression and give a form for exploration of the presenting problem' (1996: 242). In EPR terms, Luke was able to project his vision of his brain onto an inanimate object and begin to create and separate out the different areas.

Alongside this work, we worked on relaxation techniques to help Luke experience a feeling of calmness. Children with ADHD need clear structures and boundaries that promote a sense of calm. Any stimulation and excitement can add to their sense of being out of control, and therefore therapeutic work can usefully help to expand nurturing, soothing feelings.

Jernberg suggests that 'rather than challenging children to mature, you should nurture and calm the child and respond to his regressive, infantile needs' (Jernberg and Booth 2001: 193), and this can be done in a variety of ways. Luke was unsure about relaxation at first, and struggled to sit still, so we began with simple guided fantasies, with Luke sitting in one chair and me in another. I began by drawing his attention to the sound of his breathing and other sounds in the room, and gradually expanded this to include a story that emphasized being calm in a peaceful, safe place. Luke was particularly keen on the story of visiting the beach, and lying on the warm sand. Each week we practised this, extending it in length for as long as Luke could tolerate it. One day, Luke moved from the chair to sit on the pile of beanbags, and from then on he lay on a pile of cushions while I told him a story. Sometimes he covered himself with the fleece blanket and snuggled up, talking about how he felt safe and relaxed. I remained a safe distance away, in my chair, watching and talking to him in what he called my 'quiet voice'.

This was obviously an important part of the session for Luke, as it gave him the opportunity to regress to a childlike place, unobserved by his peers. We talked about how he could share these feelings with his mother, and I followed this up in discussions with her. Luke had clear memories of being cuddled by his parents when he was young, and often sought to recreate this by snuggling between them on their sofa. Luke enjoyed the sensory play, by nestling into the beanbags and wrapping himself into a soft blanket. He liked to be spoken to gently and became very still and relaxed. We thought together about how he could try to take these feelings with him into his everyday life.

Evaluation

During this period of work, Luke was finally diagnosed with ADHD and prescribed Ritalin, which he took on weekdays, before school. His teachers had already reported that he was becoming calmer, and Ritalin seemed to have an additional effect of allowing him to access the curriculum more positively. There was no noticeable difference in sessions, but Luke received more positive comments from school, which increased his self esteem.

My evaluation was based on process recordings from each session and notes taken at meetings with his parents and his school. Both Luke and his mother completed a questionnaire devised by the team to measure outcomes, in which they reported a huge improvement in self confidence and ability to concentrate. Luke said that he was not in trouble so much in school and did not get into fights in the playground.

His mother reported that Luke slept better and that the improvement in his behaviour had been noticed by the wider family. In fact Luke and his family made a visit to see other family in Australia, which would not have been possible previously, as they felt that he was now able to deal with the ordeal of the long journey.

Luke made a successful transition to High School where he continues to do well.

Whilst Ritalin in the later stages of work helped him to modify his behaviours, dramatherapy appears to have provided Luke with a place to explore his feelings and creativity. Luke was able to experience a range of holistic activities, as well as learning how to relax when under pressure. Luke used embodiment, projection and role-play in his work with me, and was able to reflect on each stage thoughtfully.

In conclusion, I believe that dramatherapy can be a useful intervention for children with ADHD, because it encourages spontaneity and creativity within the clear boundaries of a session, as well as providing a language that helps identify and manage feelings. It allows for the child to experience being someone different, through the metaphor of the drama, and helps to develop many skills that may be absorbed and developed in other areas of the child's life. It also 'enables the child to project inner conflicts onto dramatic material and this allows the problematic area to be connected to the healing possibility of drama' (Jones 2007: 154).

The therapist needs to be very clear about rules and boundaries, so that the child knows what to expect, and these can be practised with the child until they are internalized. This positive experience will also help the child to begin to have mastery over difficult emotions by promoting negotiation skills and emotional intelligence (Goleman 1996). Working together with schools, parents and medical staff can provide a wraparound service for the child in order to support them and their families and give them the best opportunity to fulfil their future potential.

References

Bannister, A. (2003) *Creative Therapies with Traumatized Children.* London: Jessica Kingsley.

Bannister, A. and Huntingdon, A. (eds.) (2002) *Communicating with Children and Adolescents. Action for Change*. London: Jessica Kingsley.

Biddulph, S. (1997) *Raising Boys. Why boys are different and how to help them become happy and well-balanced men*. London: Thorsons/Harper Collins.

Chasen, L.R. (2005) 'Spectacle and ensemble in group drama. Therapy treatment for children with ADHD and related neurological syndromes', in A.M. Weber and C. Haen (eds.), *Clinical Applications of Dramatherapy in Child and Adolescent Treatment*. East Sussex: Brunner-Routledge.

Cooper, P. and Bilton, K. (eds.) (1999) *ADHD Research, Practice and Opinion*. London: Whurr.

Gerhardt, S. (2004) *Why Love Matters. How Affection Shapes a Baby's Brain*. London: Routledge.

Goleman, D. (1996) *Emotional Intelligence. Why It Can Matter More Than IQ*. London: Bloomsbury.

Haen, C. (2005) '"Make me wanna holler." Dramatic encounters with boys from the inner city', in V. Camilleri (ed.), *Healing the Inner City Child. Creative Arts Therapies with At-Risk Youth*. London: Jessica Kingsley.

Jennings, S. (1990) *Dramatherapy with Families, Groups and Individuals, Waiting in the Wings*. London: Jessica Kingsley.

Jennings, S. (1993) *Playtherapy with Children. A Practitioner's Guide*. London: Blackwell.

Jennings, S. (ed.) (1995) *Dramatherapy with Children and Adolescents*. London: Routledge.

Jernberg, A.M. and Booth, P.B. (2001) *Theraplay. Helping Parents and Children to Build Better Relationships Through Attachment-Based Play*. London: Wiley.

Jones, P. (1996) *Drama as Therapy, Theatre as Living*. London: Routledge.

Jones, P. (2007) *Drama as Therapy. Theory, Practice and Research*. London: Routledge.

Kapalka, G.M. (2008) 'Improving self control: counselling boys with attention deficit hyperactivity disorder', in M.S. Kinselica, M. Englar-Carlson, and A.M. Horne (eds.), *Counselling Troubled Boys. A Guidebook for Professionals*. London: Routledge.

Langley, D. (2006) *An Introduction to Dramatherapy*. London: Sage.

McFarlane, P. (2005) *Dramatherapy. Developing Emotional Stability*. London: David Fulton.

Schore, A. (2003) *Affect Dysregulation and Disorders of the Self*. New York: Norton.

Williams, N.M., Zaharieva, I., Martin, A., Langley, K., Mantripagada, K., Fossdal, R., Stefansson, H., Tefansson, K., Magnusson, P., Gudmundsson, O., Gustafsson, O., Holmans, P., Owen, M. J., O'Donavan, M.C., and Thapar, A. (2010) 'Rare chromosomal deletions and duplications in attention hyperactivity disorder: A genome-wide analysis', *The Lancet* 376 (9750), 1401–1408.

6 Fear, maths, brief dramatherapy and neuroscience

Deborah E. Shine

Introduction

One of the five outcomes of the *Every Child Matters* agenda (Department for Education and Skills 2003) highlights the importance of children having emotional literacy skills if they are to make positive contributions within their communities and homes. Evidence suggests that if children are emotionally aware, they are more emotionally articulate and demonstrate greater impulse control and reasoned decision making (Elias and Weissberg 2000). Furthermore, emotional literacy skills are considered important with regards to both prevention and risk reduction in relation to children's positive emotional, psychological and social health (Adi et al. 2007; Humphrey et al. 2007; National Institute for Health and Clinical Excellence (NICE) 2008).

Schools have a key role in early identification, intervention and management of child mental health and well-being (Spratt et al. 2006; Department of Children and Families Services 2008; NICE 2008; Department of Health 2009). Consequently, schools strive nationally to promote emotional literacy through undertaking a 'whole school approach' (Department of Health and Department for Children, Schools and Families 2007). However, translating governments' initiatives from theory into practice proves challenging. Research shows that the various professionals and agencies involved do not systematically share a common professional language or culture. Subsequently, different emphasis is placed upon monitoring and achievement of outcomes, as well as defining the support needs of front-line staff (Wengrower 2001; Finney 2006; Coppock 2007).

A new approach needs establishing that is understood and compatible with all professions. It needs to be adaptable to the demands of a therapeutic and educational culture in order to be assimilated effectively into the Whole School Approach (Wengrower 2001; Finney 2006). The '6 Developmental Building Blocks' model (Banks et al. 2002, cited in Bird and Gerlach 2006; Banks et al. 2009) presented within this case study fits this purpose and was represented in *Choosing Health* (Department of Health 2004) because of its compatibility with Social and Emotional Aspects of

Learning (SEAL). This case study will illustrate how this model can be applied to a dramatherapy intervention within a mainstream school setting.

The importance of play in emotional literacy development

Conn (1997: 15) debates the relevance of dramatherapy's contribution to 'affective education and emotional support for children' in mainstream schools, suggesting emotional literacy development is better served by creative and play approaches. McFarlane (2005) emphasizes dramatherapy's potential to promote different aspects of emotional literacy development, such as self-esteem, self-confidence and self-awareness, in order to arrive at emotional stability and resilience.

Dramatherapy harnesses a child's capacity to engage in play, and evidence suggests that free play is integral to emotional, social and cognitive development (Wenner 2009). According to Wilkinson (1993), play-based therapeutic interventions have multiple functions within school settings: supporting children's neurological development, enhancing learning capacity and communication processes, as well as promoting emotional health and well-being.

Wilkinson (1993) highlights that not all children automatically learn to play, therefore the dramatherapist role models playing, both stimulating and mediating the play process (Smilansky 1968). Rike (1983) states that the shared play experience between an adult and child is crucial to both the child's future well-being and overall development. Not only is this interaction helping the child to learn about emotional self-regulation, but it also fosters the value of being in relationship with others (Howe 2005; Meldrum 2006/07).

Play and dramatherapy

Dramatherapists harness a child's capacity to engage in play, using clinical boundaries and therapeutic frameworks for the intentional purpose of healing (Jones 2007). Slade divides play into two main parts. Firstly, projective play is where the child projects the play theme 'into, onto or around objects outside' of himself, so that these objects are imbued with feeling and importance (Slade 2001: 2; Landy 1994). Secondly, personal play is when the whole child is engaged in the action: physically, emotionally and spiritually (Slade 2001). Jones (2007) presents the play–drama continuum as part of a developmental approach, the awareness of which 'can help the therapist be sensitive to shifts in functioning and to deal with them . . . via appropriate media and materials' (Irwin 1983: 150, cited in Jones 2007: 176–177). These key stages of the continuum are: sensori-motor, imitative, pretend, dramatic play and drama.

Neuroscience

Research in neurobiology can contribute to dramatherapists' understanding of play in relation to emotional regulation and Attachment Theory as well as the implications for the dramatherapist assuming the role of a reparative attachment figure (Meldrum 2006/07). By investigating neuro-physiological research, dramatherapists can reflect upon whether a child's symptomatic behaviours may be of neuro-physiological origin, rather than solely considering them as psychological, emotionally maladaptive behavioural responses, or governed by cultural and socio-economic factors (Jones 2007). The informed dramatherapist is able to consider the potential neuro-physiological impact of the therapeutic relationship and intervention, making adjustments accordingly (Meldrum 2006/07).

Developmental models

The 6 Developmental Building Blocks (Banks et al. 2009) is an integrated model of emotional literacy development, highlighting six developmental stages with their associated needs and tasks. The dramatherapist acts as emotionally responsive care-giver, providing appropriate needs-led tasks through dramatherapy to support emotional literacy development. The developmental order of the child's needs are 'Being', 'Doing', 'Thinking', 'Power and Identity', 'Structure and Skills', 'Separation and Sexuality' (Illsley Clarke and Dawson 1998). However, progression through these stages is not linear (Bird and Gerlach 2006). Unmet needs from any of these stages result in a developmental interruption, manifesting as behaviours that are often mislabelled as bad, tantrums or attention seeking.

Dramatherapy continues to develop through looking outside and beyond its own professional frame of reference, in order to evolve current best practice and the professional knowledge base (Landy 2008; Gersie 2010).

Hawkins (1984: 3) highlights the importance of dramatherapy adopting a unitary model that embraces the three aspects of creativity, learning and therapy, suggesting dramatherapy is 'a psycho-social learning process'. The 6 Developmental Building Blocks model and the accompanying 'Thrive' on-line assessment (Banks et al. 2009) takes a psycho-educational approach towards developing emotional literacy and well-being in children.

Case study: Benji

In this case study, I present a practitioner's summary of how the 6 Developmental Building Blocks model can be applied to a brief one-to-one dramatherapy intervention using free play, with a child in mainstream primary education.

The aim was to use the 6 Developmental Building Blocks model in order to:

- assess the child's developmental interruption, as indicated by the child's presenting behaviours and
- inform the course of the ongoing intervention by offering developmental stage-appropriate therapeutic interactions using dramatherapy techniques and processes.

The objective was to promote the child's emotional literacy development.

The participant, Benji, a nine-year-old boy with non-specific learning difficulties and challenging behaviour, was referred to one-to-one brief dramatherapy. He found maths difficult and distressing, which led to him banging his head repeatedly against the table. Benji needed help to find new ways of expressing his feelings at such times.

The methodology was a single clinical case study, using clinical observations of child-led projective and personal play during the dramatherapy intervention (Grainger 1999; Slade 2001). Miller et al. (2004) highlight the importance of focusing on the client's desired change in order to determine a positive therapeutic encounter and outcome. What is more, focusing on the child's perspective is in accordance with government legislation relating to the delivery of mental health services within schools (Duncan et al. 2004, 2006). The 6 Developmental Building Blocks model was used in this case study, because it specifically promotes emotional literacy development. Each of the six sessions lasted 45 minutes.

Intervention

This case study is illustrated by clinical reflections on how I responded to Benji's presenting unmet developmental needs, using dramatherapy techniques, whilst I here make reference to relevant neuro-physiological research.

Maths requires Benji's pre-frontal cortex or 'thinking' and problem-solving part of the brain to be activated. However, the pre-frontal cortex needs the positive arousal chemical dopamine to stimulate these functions, which is generated by the lower brain's SEEKING system (Panksepp 2005). If the SEEKING system is activated, Benji's pre-frontal cortex is engaged in learning processes due to the stimulation of curiosity and motivation (Sunderland 2006). One way to activate the SEEKING system is through creative play, such as promoted within dramatherapy (Sunderland 2006).

However, a critical and unpredictable response would automatically trigger stress-inducing chemicals (cortisol and adrenaline) to flood Benji's brain. This would shut down neural pathways leading to or from the pre-frontal cortex, inhibiting Benji's ability to engage in learning processes (Sunderland 2006). When this happened, Benji would also experience a neuro-physiological surge to discharge pent-up physical energy, which he often expressed through self-harm.

My therapeutic intention was to develop Benji's ability and tolerance for 'thinking' by introducing it as a pleasurable symbolic experience where there was no right or wrong way. Therefore, every dramatherapy session started with child-led play, thus ensuring Benji did not experience failure and shame, which was often triggered when he engaged in 'thinking' processes such as maths. This is highly relevant because shame neurophysiologically inhibits the SEEKING system (Sunderland 2006).

Without realizing it, Benji playfully took risks, made decisions, problem-solved and reflected upon consequences as he explored, developed and initiated creative play in dramatherapy. Often Benji resorted to doing things in the expected way, once he had creatively explored all other options. In the sessions, Benji's diverse approach was not perceived as contrariness. Instead it became a source of inspiration and esteem, enabling Benji to explore the thinking processes of cause and effect. The activities Benji developed became progressively more complex and interactive, as his curiosity in our therapeutic relationship grew. I consciously maintained an attitude of PACE – playfulness, acceptance, curiosity and empathy (Hughes 2007). My intention was to become Benji's psycho-biological regulator, identifying and responding to his emotional and developmental needs, mirroring his responses and naming feelings. I also offered physically interactive activities to support Benji's need to discharge energy. Consequently, Benji naturally integrated me into his play.

In school, the adults around Benji often found it difficult to remain emotionally responsive when faced with his escalating behaviour, possibly because they also felt failure, shame and blame. However, by remaining self-aware, the dramatherapist is professionally equipped to recognize such counter-transference (Landy 1994) and subsequently to self-soothe and self-regulate by engaging her own pre-frontal cortex during the therapeutic encounter. Benji would learn to regulate his own feelings most effectively if he was in relationships with others who are able to self-regulate and self-soothe (Meldrum 2006/07).

Benji's desire to explore and relate remained overriding themes throughout the sessions, shaping Benji's ritual interactive activities. Landy (1994: 69) describes the anthropological practice of ritual as 'symbolic action repeated in a prescribed way', for the purposes of maintaining 'the status quo', affirming 'a common bond between members' which helps 'to defend . . . against danger'. He emphasizes that as rituals are expressions of healing and performance 'through acts of imagination', they are 'excellent sources for drama therapy' (1994: 71). The combination of exploration, ownership and ritual appeared to make the therapeutic encounter and 'thinking' more predictable and safe for Benji, whilst enabling us to discover the 'play language' of our therapeutic relationship (Jones 2007). Focusing on practical tasks moderates the intensity of an interaction, helping to reduce anxiety for children such as Benji who have attachment issues (Geddes 2006).

Jones (2007: 277) highlights the importance of the dramatherapist grounding the client's relationship practically between their own ritual and dramatherapy within three key areas: reproduction, reframing and reworking of incomplete or problematic ritual experiences, 'using ritual forms to deal with client's material . . . which can usefully be considered or analysed within a ritual framework'.

Initially, Benji's 'doing' needs were met by me delivering a running commentary of his ritual explorations around the room and equipment without any interpretation. Benji soon started to focus his attention on the solitary exploration of single objects. Then Benji initiated sporadic interaction by showing me his chosen object. He developed this interaction further by asking me to pass him specific objects. Soon he engaged me in reciprocal play. Benji's needs for solitary exploration accompanied by my verbal commentary became a child-led ritual at the beginning of every session.

Benji appeared to experience an increasing sense of agency through his actions both in relation to the space and our relationship. As dramatherapist, I was responsible for reinforcing Benji's 'being' needs through regulating experiences so they were manageable, offering Benji unconditional positive regard. I attended to both Benji's physical and emotional comfort and I made available sensory mediums such as sand play, cushions and coloured fabric.

Benji's eagerness and capacity to instigate reciprocal ritual play evolved over the sessions alongside our relationship. As a result, Benji developed rules, order and narrative. One ritual story Benji evolved through projective free play using small objects (Landy 1994; Slade 2001), and involved two characters he called Snake and Alien playing hide and seek. Over time it appeared to reflect Benji's increasing ability to tolerate his ambivalence towards our relationship (Landy 1994). In the first two sessions, Snake (animated by me under Benji's instructions) would seek out and kill Alien (animated by Benji). Whilst I acted out Benji's instructions, I introduced empathy through Snake expressing remorse. Gradually Benji evolved the ritual encounter into Alien performing death-defying leaps, seeking to be chased and eventually caught and tickled by Snake rather than being murdered. Landy (1994: 153) highlights that as objects are 'the most abstract and distanced' of the projective devices, they help the dramatherapist to discover 'how the child sees himself and what he needs from significant others'. Through the course of the sessions, Benji's experience of attachment appeared to change from fear of annihilation to the joy of interdependency, as depicted in his play between Snake and Alien.

Gersie (1997: 4) highlights the value of story making to emotional literacy development, as a collaborative process of 'storied doing', facilitating emotional expression, reflection upon feelings and thoughts, as well as the reinterpretation of 'action, statements and practices'. She describes this as a therapeutic-educational process, where it is crucial that the damatherapist also engages fully in the play process (Gersie 1987). Bannister (2008: 19) describes how children and the archetypes and symbolism used within dramatherapy comfortably co-habit the 'third space' of play.

Through reciprocal play, Benji started to express, explore and tolerate the differences between contrary and co-habiting emotions, such as anger, sadness and joy (Gerhardt 2004).

As dramatherapist, I also had a neuro-physiological role. As the processes of thinking and learning occur within the pre-frontal cortex, their development is determined by Benji receiving consistent and emotionally responsive care-giving, particularly at times of fear and distress. Its transformative potential is represented in Benji's growing tolerance of his ambivalence towards attachment, as depicted in his 'alien and snake' story. A combination of physical and emotional reassurance, non-verbal mirroring and predictable responses from the dramatherapist intend to release stress-reducing chemicals (i.e. oxytocin) into the brain, stimulating the development of neural pathways to and from the pre-frontal cortex to the lower mammalian and reptilian brains. As a result, Benji's fight–flight responses to fear and distress, triggered in the lower mammalian brain, were replaced by a sense of well-being (Sunderland 2006). This was evidenced by Benji's increased neuro-physiological capacity to emotionally self-regulate, to talk about feelings and to problem-solve as well as to understand cause and effect (Sunderland 2006). As these sessions progressed, this transformative process was depicted symbolically and therapeutically by Benji making adjustments to the ritual story's ending. Through dramatherapy, Benji engaged in the reparative experiences of 'second chance learning' (Winnicott 1965).

There was evidence to suggest that Benji progressed through stages relating to the 6 Developmental Building Blocks model that had similarities to Jones' (2007) play-drama continuum. In Benji's first session, erratic butterfly behaviour suggested a developmental interruption at the 'doing' stage. He randomly moved around the space, picking up objects, only to put them down rapidly. This solitary play resembled the 'sensorimotor play' stage (2007: 178). Benji's 'doing' needs had to be addressed through dramatherapy if he was to move on to the next developmental stage of 'thinking'. Only then would Benji be neuro-physiologically able to engage his pre-frontal cortex in the 'thinking' processes required for activities such as maths.

Evaluation

The following evaluation procedures emerged from Benji's free play within the dramatherapy sessions. From the first session Benji spontaneously introduced ritual activities that were then adopted as child-centred evaluation tools in each consecutive session. I referred to these child-led procedures as 'Feeling Faces' and 'Animal Sand Prints'. These child-led rituals also served to promote Benji's sense of agency and self-esteem within the therapeutic encounter and evaluation process.

'Feeling Faces' consisted of a selection of individual circles, each showing a facial expression depicting a specific emotion. At the start of the first session, Benji initiated picking out faces that showed me how he was feeling. Consequently, at the beginning and end of every subsequent session, Benji was invited to choose 'Feeling Faces' to show his feeling states at those points in time, developing his emotional awareness and literacy.

As sessions progressed, Benji selected increasing numbers and ranges of 'Feeling Faces'. He started choosing opposing feelings simultaneously. He commented how his feelings changed throughout the session, suggesting growing self-awareness, an expanding emotional vocabulary, as well as an increased ability to tolerate ambivalence and self-regulate. Benji also spontaneously evaluated his dramatherapy experience by telling me how it made him feel.

'Animal Sand Prints' emerged when Benji spontaneously expressed his 'doing' needs by pressing animal objects into a wet sandtray, during sensori-motor play. This child-led ritual evolved from Benji meeting his 'being' needs through exploring the sensorial sand. As sessions progressed, Benji engaged me in increasingly complex reciprocal interactive play whereby we used actions and sounds to describe the chosen imprinted object. This process parallels progression through 'imitative play' to 'pretend play' (Jones 2007). Benji also introduced words, problem-solving, structure and rules into this activity, suggesting his developmental interruptions and needs were being progressively met.

I offered the 'being' task of unconditional positive regard during Benji's spontaneous sensory sand play. Benji then started to randomly place and bury small figures under the sand, expressing his 'doing' needs. I offered the 'doing' task of verbal commentary to accompany his actions. Soon Benji asked me to guess the animal he had imprinted in the sand, as if I were to role-model 'thinking'. This was the first time in our encounter that there was a right or wrong answer and it was Benji who was introducing the concept to our play. Benji's previous experiences of 'thinking' about right or wrong answers were associated with feelings of shame, blame and abandonment, particularly in maths. Benji witnessed me guessing and surviving without shame. Soon, Benji was eager to take on the guessing role, expressing his 'thinking' needs.

As sessions progressed, Benji continued to initiate this ritual activity and adapt it further, suggesting an increased ability to identify and meet his own 'thinking' needs (Bird and Gerlach 2006; Jones 2007). Guessing appeared increasingly self-rewarding for Benji as he explored all possible ways to describe the animal object, other than by its obvious name. We mimed the animal's call, walk and what it ate, through 'dramatic play' (Jones 2007: 182). Benji was fully engaged in 'thinking' and loving every moment. His sense of agency, self-worth and self-esteem grew, meeting 'power and identity needs' within a supportive dramatherapy encounter (Bird and Gerlach 2006).

Prior to dramatherapy, Benji was a solitary child, who was rarely seen playing. Once engaged in dramatherapy, Benji was not only observed engaging school peers in play, but was also inventing, repeating and evolving his own relational games. This demonstrated Benji was transferring newly acquired skills from therapy into school. This process also suggests that through the course of dramatherapy, Benji was generating and internalizing additional significant and pleasurable attachment memories and associations, within the hippocampus part of his brain, corresponding to RIGS – Representations of Interactions that have been Generalized outlined by Stern (2000).

Third party feedback was given at the end of the intervention by Benji's teaching staff and mother. They all perceived developments in Benji's emotional literacy and well-being. At school, instead of standing alone at break times, Benji was observed frequently playing with a new, small, group of friends. He spoke with trusted adults when experiencing difficult feelings, rather than withdrawing. In maths, Benji's self-harming behaviour significantly reduced. At home, Benji's mother reported that he often told her how much he enjoyed the dramatherapy sessions.

Conclusion

This case study demonstrates how current research in neuroscience can inform dramatherapy practice and highlight its benefits within a school.

Firstly, the child's presenting behaviours can be de-pathologized and considered as symptomatic of temporary hormone imbalances, resulting from developmental interruptions. Secondly, sharing such understanding with other multi-agency professionals can impact upon their perception of the child's presenting behaviour, enabling them to review the child's support needs accordingly. Thirdly, the dramatherapist can consider and investigate the potential neuro-physiological impact of the dramatherapy relationship, techniques and processes upon the child's needs and behaviours throughout the course of the intervention.

Furthermore, the 6 Developmental Building Blocks model appears compatible with dramatherapy's developmental approach and the play–drama continuum (Jones 2007). Grounded in neuroscience, it can inform and shape the initial and ongoing dramatherapy assessment and intervention, responding to the developmental needs of the individual child. This supports the dramatherapist's understanding of the impact of neuro-physiological processes upon a child's capacity to engage in play and learning, which is highly pertinent to dramatherapists working within education. This model also provides a common language accessible to clinicians, educationalists and social care professionals.

Within this case study, Benji's participation in dramatherapy coincided with a significant reduction in self-harm behaviour, suggesting he was more able to emotionally self-soothe and self-regulate. Teaching staff and his parent perceived significant changes in Benji's emotional and social behaviour with an increased ability to engage in rewarding relationships. This suggested significant developments in emotional literacy. Dramatherapy techniques and processes were used to give Benji manageable developmental stage-sensitive experiences, fostered within an emotionally responsive relationship. Benji appeared to find dramatherapy both an accessible and reparative experience, where he experienced the unexpected rewards of thinking and learning alongside play and positive attachment.

I have been applying the 6 Developmental Building Blocks model within my short- and long-term client dramatherapy practice since 2007, after undertaking training with Sowelu Associates (Bird and Gerlach 2006). Subsequently I have found its application has enhanced my understanding of emotional literacy development, enriched my clinical practice and facilitated dialogue with multi-agency child-care professionals, including teaching staff.

References

Adi, Y., Killoran, A., Janmohamed, K., and Stewart-Brown, S. (2007) *Systematic review of the effectiveness of interventions to promote mental well-being in primary schools. Universal approaches which do not focus on violence or bullying*, University of Warwick, Report 1, www.nice.org.uk/nicemedia/pdf/MentalWellbeingWarwickUniReview.pdf (Accessed 6 May 2010).

Banks, J., Bird, J., Gerlach, L., and Lovelock, J. (2009) *Thrive Fronting the Challenge (ftc) Projects: Emotional Development for Well-being and Learning*, http://www.thriveftc.com (Accessed 19 May 2010).

Bannister, A. (2008) *Creative Therapies with Traumatised Children*. London: Jessica Kingsley.

Bird, J. and Gerlach, L. (2006) *Certificate in Emotional Literacy for Children*. Training Literature, Sowelu Associates (E-mail: EmLitSW@aol.com), in association with The Institute for Arts in Therapy & Education, London, http://www.artspsychotherapy.org.

Conn, C. (1997) 'Schools and dramatherapy: A closer look at the curriculum', *Dramatherapy, Journal of the British Association of Dramatherapists*, 19 (1), 15–21.

Coppock, V. (2007) 'It's good to talk! A multidimensional qualitative study of the effectiveness of emotional literacy work in schools', *Children and Society*, 21, 405–419.

Department for Education and Skills (2003) *Every Child Matters*. London: HMSO.

Department of Children and Families Services (2008) *Targeted Mental Health in Schools Project – Using the evidence to inform your approach: a practical guide to head teachers and commissioners*. DCSF-00784-2008. Nottingham: DCFS Publications.

Department of Health (2004) 'Children and young people – Starting on the right path', in *Choosing Health: Making healthy choices easier*. CM6374. London: Crown Publishers.

Department of Health (2009) *Healthy Lives, Brighter Futures. The strategy for children and young people's health*. 285374a. London: Crown Publishers.

Department of Health and Department for Children, Schools and Families (2007)

Introduction to the National Healthy Schools Programme. NHSP Introduction v.2/08/07/ICE6055. London: Crown Publishers.

Duncan, B.L., Miller, S.D., and Sparks, J.A. (2004) *The Heroic Client: A revolutionary way to improve effectiveness through client-directed, outcome-informed therapy*. San Francisco: Jossey Bass Wiley.

Duncan, B.L., Sparks, J.A., Miller, S.D., Bohanske, R.T., and Claud, D.A. (2006) 'Giving youth a voice: a preliminary study of the reliability and validity of a brief outcome measure for children, adolescents, and caretakers', *Journal of Brief Therapy* 5 (2),

Elias, M.J. and Weissberg, R.P. (2000) 'Primary prevention: educational approaches to enhance social and emotional learning', *Journal of School Health*, 70, 186–190.

Finney, D. (2006) 'Stretching the boundaries: schools as therapeutic agents in mental health. Is it a realistic proposition?' *Pastoral Care*, September, 22–27.

Geddes, H. (2006) *Attachment in the Classroom*. London: Worth.

Gerhardt, S. (2004) *Why Love Matters*. London: Routledge.

Gersie, A. (1987) 'Dramatherapy and play', in S. Jennings (ed.), *Dramatherapy: theory and practice for teachers and clinicians*. London: Croom Helm.

Gersie, A. (1997) *Reflections on Therapeutic Storymaking*. London: Jessica Kingsley.

Gersie, A. (2010) Personal, written communication about the history of EPR/Dramatherapy. 7 April.

Grainger, R. (1999) *Researching the Arts Therapists. A Dramatherapist's Perspective*. London: Jessica Kingsley.

Hawkins, P. (1984) 'Dramatherapy: In search of wholeness. A reply to Sue Jennings Models of Practice in Dramatherapy', *Dramatherapy, Journal of the British Association of Dramatherapists*, 8 (1), 3–7.

Howe, D. (2005) *Child Abuse and Neglect*. Hampshire: Palgrave Macmillan.

Hughes, D. (2007) *Attachment Focused Family Therapy*. London: Norton.

Humphrey, N., Curran, A., Morris, E., Farrell, P., and Woods, K. (2007) 'Emotional intelligence and education: A critical review', *Educational Psychology*, 27 (2), 235–254.

Illsley Clarke, J. and Dawson, C. (1998) *Growing Up Again*. Minnesota: Hazelden, 2nd edition.

Irwin, E.C. (1983) 'The diagnostic and therapeutic use of pretend play', in C.E. Shaefer and K.J. O'Connor (eds.) *The Handbook of Play Therapy*. New York: Wiley.

Jones, P. (2007) *Drama as Therapy: Theory, Practice and Research*. New York: Routledge, 2nd edition.

Landy, R.J. (1994) *Drama Therapy: Concepts, Theories and Practices*. Springfield IL: Charles C. Thomas, 2nd edition.

Landy, R.J. (2008) 'The dramatic world view revisited – reflections on the roles taken and played by young children and adolescents', *Dramatherapy, Journal of the British Association of Dramatherapists*, 30 (2), 3–13.

McFarlane, P. (2005) *Dramatherapy: Developing Emotional Stability*. London: David Fulton.

Meldrum, B. (2006/07) 'The drama of attachment', *Dramatherapy, Journal of the British Association of Dramatherapists*, 28 (3), 10–20.

Miller, S.D., Duncan, B.L., and Hubble, M.A. (2004) 'Beyond integration: triumph of outcome over process in clinical practice', *Psychotherapy in Australia*, 10 (2), 2–19.

National Institute for Health and Clinical Excellence (2008) *Promoting Children's Social and Emotional Well-being in Primary education.* NICE Public Health Guidance 12. London: NICE.

Panksepp, J. (2005) *Affective Neuroscience.* Oxford: Oxford University Press.

Rike, E. (1983) *A Research Design: Review of literature in the commonalities of creative drama, language, communication and creative thinking.* Unpublished manuscript, University of Tennessee, Knoxville, cited in J.A. Wilkinson (1993) *The Symbolic Dramatic Play – Literacy Connection*, Needham Heights: Ginn Press.

Slade, P. (2001) *Child Play.* London: Jessica Kingsley, 2nd impression.

Smilansky, S. (1968) *The Effects of Socio-dramatic Play on Disadvantaged Pre-school Children.* New York: John Wiley and Sons.

Spratt, J., Shucksmith, J., Philip, K., and Watson, C. (2006) 'Part of who we are as a school should include responsibility for well-being', *Pastoral Care*, September, 14–21.

Stern, D. (2000) *The Interpersonal World of the Infant.* New York: Basic Books.

Sunderland, M. (2006) *The Science of Parenting.* London: Dorling Kindersley.

Wengrower, H. (2001) 'Arts therapies in educational settings: an intercultural encounter', *The Arts in Psychotherapy*, 28 (2), 109–115.

Wenner, M. (2009) 'The serious need to play', *Scientific American Mind*, 20, 1.

Wilkinson, J.A. (1993) *The Symbolic Dramatic Play – Literacy Connection.* Needham Heights: Ginn Press.

Winnicott, D.W. (1965) *The Maturational Process and Facilitating Environment.* London: Kamac Books.

7 Violence and laughter: how school-based dramatherapy can go beyond behaviour management for boys at risk of exclusion from school

Dolmen Domikles

Introduction

This chapter explores some of the opportunities that working as a dramatherapist in the role of Primary Mental Health Worker (PMHW) offers within a secondary school. Helping young people with a particular range of difficulties to survive in mainstream education, where they are often not able to be helped by conventional child and adolescent mental health services (CAMHS), is an important aspect of this work.

Some reflections on the limitations of traditional CAMHS teams in helping serious behaviour problems at school are included. The focus of the chapter is a group of young people with traumatic histories and family lives, who are frequently excluded from school because of their angry and violent outbursts. However, often they do not access therapeutic services. The existing dramatherapy literature on this subject will be looked at. Finally a brief dramatherapy intervention is described, with a conclusion about possibilities for future work.

Some limitations of traditional CAMHS in working with school exclusion

Overwhelming demand has often resulted in CAMHS needing to limit their interventions to more severe cases, which it can be convenient to identify by medical diagnosis. Even though individual practitioners may holistically view young people in emotional crisis, CAMHS commissioners' demands may require them to find non-holistic definitions to direct their service to the cases needing their more specialized skills.

Another limiting factor for children getting help from CAMHS based in NHS clinics is their dependence on their parents to bring them to appointments. If their parents fail to bring them, children cannot be helped by a traditional clinic-based CAMHS. Often work with the family would be more successful than meeting with the young person alone, but sometimes, as soon as there is the first suggestion that the child's problems may have some connection with experiences within the family, the child is never seen again at the clinic.

A third problem can be that some adolescent boys in particular who have behaviour problems do not respond well to verbally-based therapies, because of difficulties with emotional literacy.

These factors mean that school staff can feel left alone in trying to provide education for students with very traumatic histories, whose behaviour is causing repeated and eventually permanent exclusion. As this chapter shows, school-based dramatherapy is a medium that can sometimes overcome this problem.

Basing therapeutic services within schools is a response to at least some of these barriers. Once a parent or carer has given permission, a professional working in a school can talk to the child, ask for his agreement and ensure their appointments are kept.

Dramatherapy within primary mental health work in CAMHS

In my work as a CAMHS Primary Mental Health Worker (Health Advisory Service 1995) I have developed a dramatherapy practice. As the post has developed, part of my work involves offering interventions to two students at any one time in a particular secondary school. Referrals came initially from local GPs who had been visited by the parents who had worries about their children who attended the school. I worked with the families, or worked individually with their children. In terms of the changes wished for by the students, these interventions often seemed successful. Dramatherapy was one of the approaches used.

However, various staff in the school expressed the need for help with other boys they felt desperately concerned about. These boys were highly distressed, losing their temper, getting into fights with other students, being rude to teachers and walking out of lessons. This behaviour would lead necessarily to exclusions. As the days of exclusion totted up, permanent exclusion would unavoidably follow. Admission to other schools could be followed by serial exclusions. It is known that boys with this educational history can suffer from severe disadvantages and poorer life outcomes later on (Social Policy Research Unit 2004: 2).

Often when these young people were referred to CAMHS the parents either did not attend, or attended once or twice and then no more. It was becoming clear to me that there was a group of young people at the school who were living in family situations that were causing them great distress. Often their problems were noticed as soon as they entered the school system. Family relationships were unstable, featuring abandonment, emotional neglect, and ongoing conflict. Most boys had witnessed domestic violence. It was possible that early attachment to their carer(s) had been insecure. The school pastoral team were desperate to help these boys, and asked me to intervene.

Exploring the evidence base

In my search for the evidence, I noticed a lack of models of previous work that seemed to address this kind of problem. There was a great deal of literature about 1:1 or group dramatherapy or play therapy with children who were known to be victims of abuse (Bannister 1995, 2003; Cattanach 1992a, 1992b; James et al. 2005). There were equally some writings about groupwork with young people, generally boys, with behaviour difficulties in school (Quibell 2010). Emunah (1995) has written about similar groups in a psychiatric setting. Since this work was carried out, Christensen (2010) describes individual work with an excluded 11-year-old boy in a Student Support Unit in a secondary school. I was interested in trying to offer a solution that within dramatherapy might safely address some of the traumas underlying behaviour that did not appear to have been clearly identified or worked with. I noticed how at school it can be easy to talk about behaviour problems ('conduct disorder' or 'oppositional-defiant disorder' being the psychiatric equivalent). In fact there may be a history of traumatic episodes or family dysfunction which explains the behaviour.

A model called Developmental Transformations (DvT) was developed in the US, and has been successfully used with various client groups, including children who have suffered abuse (James et al. 2005). DvT is a very well-researched and well-documented approach, taught in the US, Netherlands and Israel. With DvT:

> The therapist attempts to reveal aspects of the client's inner experience through complete involvement with emergent patterns in the client's play.
> The therapist must join the client in the playspace.
> The therapist (serves) as the client's playobject.
> (The therapist) sacrifices privilege, control, or even self-definition.
>
> (Johnson et al. 1996: 297)

Johnson's method involves rapid transformations within the scene (Johnson 1991: 290). This was to be my approach.

Introduction to 'Jake'

The case accepted from the Head of Year 8 was of a 12-year-old boy, here called Jake, who was at risk of permanent exclusion. He was apparently angry and wound-up in lessons, and lashed out at other boys. He had difficulty expressing his feelings. The CAMHS records showed that he had been first referred to CAMHS at the age of 8. It was reported that his 6-year-old brother had a diagnosis of attention deficit hyperactivity disorder (ADHD) and autism, and that Jake was often woken by his brother hitting him. They would fight, and frequently hurt each other. At school Jake was said to be aggressive and attention-seeking. The family did not attend their appointment following that referral. Jake was re-referred subsequently, and was seen with his mother at the age of 10. His mother disclosed that Jake's father had been violent against her, once injuring her face. Aggression between the brothers was continuing. School reported that Jake presented as 'very disturbed and angry', 'verbally and physically aggressive to both adults and children'. Those who work in city schools know that this scenario is more commonly witnessed than talked about. Jake's mother said that he hit out because people were annoying, and she had always 'taught him to stick up for himself'. She requested anger management for Jake, however at his assessment, Jake refused to say a word and as a result the CAMHS worker felt unable to help him. At that time he had also just been referred to the Behaviour Support Service. Jake was discharged from CAMHS.

Jake's problems were deepseated. The traumatizing effects of domestic violence are well known (Kolbo et al. 1996). If the violence was sufficiently frequent, it is possible that Jake's mother's response to his early attachment needs was affected, leading to insecure attachment. This was being compounded at present by constant extremely violent conflict with his brother with special needs, who would require much of the family's attention. It seemed that his mother was not able to empathize with Jake's needs. Maybe his inability to verbalize his feelings or problems might be related to a general difficulty with emotional literacy in the home. Even though I was aware of the limitations of a short-term intervention, I decided to respond to the concerns of the school as there seemed sufficient evidence that dramatherapy could help him to change his behaviour.

First meeting with Jake and his mother

I made an appointment to meet with Jake and his mother. Jake also had a stepfather, whom I did not meet. His mother described Jake getting angry and not listening. She said that he would shout, kick and slam the door, but not hit out or break things. He would sometimes be dragged to his room by his stepfather, and would apparently calm down in 5–20 minutes. Jake's mother felt that he had a problem, and hoped that anger management could help him. Neither Jake nor his mother were able to suggest any reasons for Jake's angry behaviour. I asked Jake how he would like his life to be different and he said that he would like to be able to stop getting so angry. He also said he would like to meet with me to try some dramatherapy.

I was aware that this assessment was a little limited, but I firmly felt that the previous history collected by CAMHS, the present situation that I was aware of from the school, and the request from both Jake and his mother augured well for dramatherapy with Jake. Jake's mother was obviously reluctant to consider family dynamics that might be causing Jake's anger.

There was a sufficient mandate to start work with Jake. My standard short-term intervention of six sessions was offered to him.

Precautionary comments about the inner processes of the dramatherapist

For those who are less acquainted with the dramatherapeutic process, some preliminary explanation is necessary. Children who have experienced violence are often unable to express to others in words their feelings about what they have experienced. Unconsciously, they try to let other people know how they feel by making them feel the same thing, through their behaviour. That is why school staff can have feelings of anger, hopelessness, inadequacy, confusion and despair in relation to these children. The children are projecting their own feelings into the teachers. The staff members may find their professionalism challenged, because teachers are not expected to have these feelings (chapter 14 in this book, by Kelly and Bruck, gives a model for staff sharing for this kind of supportive staff work).

The aim of dramatherapy is to enable the young person to project these feelings into the drama, and – depending on the model of dramatherapy used – onto the dramatherapist in role. This can provide relief to the client, and the chance to come to terms with these feelings and experiences. In the DvT model the dramatherapist needs to be able to experience all these feelings him/herself in role. This is part of the work and why dramatherapists take their work to supervision, to keep the work with their clients safe.

In psychodynamic psychotherapy the client may project these intolerable feelings into the therapist. The therapist notices these feelings within him/herself. This is known as 'countertransference' (Brown and Pedder 1979: 64–66). The therapist reflects on what these countertransference feelings tell him about the inner state of the client. In dramatherapy, as well as the feelings projected into the drama and the dramatherapist in role, the dramatherapist may also experience these uncomfortable feelings within himself as the therapist. This process is a normal experience for a dramatherapist/psychotherapist who is trained to cope with them. A dramatherapist cannot help a client unless they are prepared to join them and share some of their world. As chapter 14 explains in more detail, supervision enables therapists to stand back from their work and look with their supervisor at the feelings this brings up in them, and to think about these in connection with the client's difficulties.

In contrast, the teaching profession is expected to work very differently with difficult feelings which come up in the classroom.

The reader may find some of the following material puzzling and worrying. This resonates with the world of the young person. The next section shows the criteria for this work.

Safety

Physical safety as well as mental safety is paramount in this work. Dramatherapy, which may involve the use of physical contact, is an ideal intervention (British Association of Dramatherapists Code of Conduct 2005). I have worked as a dramatherapist in CAMHS for the last nine years, and for the last four years since this case a significant part of my caseload has been work with violent boys. Pretend playfighting within the drama has been introduced by the boys in a majority of those cases, and every time has turned out to have some effect in helping them in learning to control their violence in real life. Fathers all over the world playfight with their sons in order to 'have fun, get noisy, even get angry and, at the same time, *know when to stop*' (Biddulph 1997: 74). Playfighting offers an opportunity to show care for the other within the playfight. In my practice, and without exception, clear boundaries are always set at the outset, and this ensures the safety of the work.

As well as this, dramatherapy works with an emphasis on deroling, which ensures a safe return to class. Deroling is an established dramatherapy technique, which ensures that, at the end of the session, the client leaves the dramatic material in the dramatherapy space, and further, that any destructive dramatic roles can be safely played within the therapy, without the danger they might be re-enacted by the client in real life.

Early dramatherapy sessions with Jake

Session I

In our first session, Jake responded well to some initial 'getting to know you' type games, although as before, when asked for more details about when and how he got angry at school or at home, Jake became monosyllabic, and became listless. This contrasted with the energy and humour he showed when playing with small puppets, when he was asked to choose puppets to represent his family. The tableau quickly developed into an endless battle between family members. Despite the grim imagery, there were humorous moments. Jake was obviously comfortable with using his imagination. He had a sense of symbolism, and he was able clearly to make the link between the play and reality. This felt like a propitious first session.

Session II

The session began with a game of throwing and catching a beanbag, following Jenning's idea of using embodied activity in entering dramatic work (Jennings 1990: 10–11). Jake noticed Frank, a knitted doll, a clown/tramp character, whom I had placed in a sitting and watching position in the room. From this moment I was able to draw Jake into dramatic improvisation, similar to the DvT model, but adapted, in that DvT uses no props at all. In this improvisation we had Frank as a third character in the drama, animated by either Jake or me. Frank was animated by me to take on the role of a badly behaved, violent boy. Jake, in the role of a parent, punished Frank by shutting him in a suitcase, from which he would 'escape' to behave badly again. Even though the story included violence, where a knitted doll would be animated by one of us to 'attack' the other, and the parent's 'punishment' was quite unpleasant, the drama had a cartoon quality, where these actions became funny. There was much energy and laughter in the drama, even though I felt it very likely that the material related to Jake's very difficult experiences in real life. The model of improvisation I follow is influenced by the work of Keith Johnstone (1981).

Session III: 'Hamming it up'

The third session started with Jake recapitulating the story of Frank 'attacking' each of us. I noticed Jake's evident pleasure and excitement in seeing me acting hurt, when he animated the woolly doll to 'hit' me. I hammed it up, increased my shouting, groaning and writhing. Jake's eyes opened wide, and he laughed. Jake animated Frank to attack me more.

The action then transformed as Jake picked up the tiny grandfather figurine he had chosen to represent me in our first session and began to torment this figure. When I reacted myself in role to the pain he had inflicted on the figurine, he said, 'Voodoo!' and laughed. When he threw the figure, I flew across the room. He did different things to the figure, seeming to experiment what he could direct me to do dramatically. I did my best to imitate whatever the puppet was forced to do. Then he found the figure representing himself, Jake, in session I, and he invited me to playfully torment him in turn. Jake then had fun being 'thrown' around the room. Next, he animated Frank to throw both of our figures around the room, and we both had fun flying around and acting crashing against the walls.

Jake and I were developing a dramatic language where violence and trauma could be represented between us in a way that was non-threatening to Jake, because it was in the playspace. The humour, and the evident care we each took not to harm the other, made it safe. Dramatherapy offers the opportunity to re-experience past trauma through creating the right distance from the trauma, called the 'aesthetic distance' by Landy (1992: 99), whereby 'the individual is capable of feeling, without fear of being overwhelmed by the emotion'. Aesthetic distance and developing a dramatic language ensure safety in the therapeutic space.

Session IV

Amid the familiar motifs that we had developed together, Jake and I enacted a complex story. He took on a succession of roles. First he acted himself, and then successively his mother, his father, his granddad, his grandma, and finally an ancestor. Each of his characters announced who they were, and said they were going to beat me up. I noticed that now Jake felt safe enough to act fighting against me himself, in role, although without any direct physical contact. He was rapidly miming the blows, stopping them before they hit me, and within the 'as if' quality of dramatherapy I reacted strongly as if I had been hit. The drama was energizing. In between each of these scenes, Jake would become himself, sitting in the chair, maintaining that the previous scene had never happened.

At the end of the session, I commented that the boy at the beginning of the story had no chance of not being violent, when violence went on so much in his life. He looked down and grunted listlessly. Even though he had no words to express it, I felt that Jake was cognitively processing his traumatic experiences, and maybe making a comment about how his own violent patterns of behaviour had come about.

Reflections on the first six sessions

The most accurate way to evaluate the effectiveness or otherwise of this intervention was to look with the team for change in Jake's behaviour because Jake's limited verbal expression meant I was unable to gain specific feedback on what he might feel was helpful. But he did agree that he felt dramatherapy was helping.

Jake's pastoral assistant reported that when a fight occurred, Jake was now releasing his hold of his adversary when asked. He also was now seeking her out to help him calm down after an angry episode. Even though violent episodes were still occurring, this seemed to be a significant change in Jake. The Deputy Head was keen for me to work further with Jake. Her office was next door to the dramatherapy room. She could hear the noise. She told me that she had the sense that this work was exactly what Jake needed. My clinical supervisor and my manager were both supportive of this work continuing. I asked Jake if he would like another six sessions, and he said yes.

Evaluation of the outcome of the intervention: further improvement in Jake's behaviour

At the end of the twelfth session, Jake and the school reported further improvement in his behaviour. He was losing his temper less. The school had previously arranged for Jake to spend some time at the Pupil Referral Unit, until near the end of the school year. There he could have some time away from the boys he had habitually fought with at school. In September, when Jake returned to school, it was noticed that he was not getting into fights at all. This change persisted. I wondered whether there had been other changes in his family environment. A year later, I met with Jake briefly, to ask his permission to publish this material, and asked him what had changed in his situation at home. He said that nothing else had changed in his family situation. When asked what had helped him to improve things at school, Jake said 'The drama'. It is interesting to wonder therefore if the fact that this took place in school meant that it had a direct effect on Jake's behaviour in school. Had the same work taken place outside school, would this outcome have been the same?

At the time of writing, Jake is in his first year of college. He has managed to remain at school ever since this intervention, without fighting or getting into trouble for angry outbursts. Significant difficulties at home were reported in his last year, but Jake's education at school was not threatened. His mother reported to me recently that he obtained good GCSE results, and is now doing well at college. He now lives with his grandmother.

So in terms of the initial aim of trying to help Jake to avoid exclusion and complete his education, the intervention was successful. It is also likely that Jake's quality of life at least at school was significantly better. In the opinion of the School Deputy Head in charge of the Pastoral Team, for those children whose family life is not stable, school represents a safe haven. Therefore, having a stable school life is of extra importance to those children.

Reflections on what worked

There is evidence here that this intervention was effective. It is useful to try to understand firstly why it was effective, and secondly whether or not this approach may have been more effective than other approaches.

As mentioned, Developmental Transformations, a dramatherapeutic method originally explored and written about by David Read Johnson, provides a theoretical framework for understanding this intervention. My method of working described above, and developed since, has some parallels and similarities with DvT. Having had opportunities to train with David Read Johnson on several occasions, I am now part of an ongoing DvT practice group being trained by him. The themes that Jake created through this work revealed aspects of his world. Themes included the casual and systematic causing of pain, cruelty, punishment, confusion, disorientation, guilt, shame, accusation, humiliation and madness. James et al. (2005), in their account of individual DvT-based dramatherapy with an eight-year-old abused boy, describe how for the first six months the stories consisted mainly of the boy 'hurting' and 'killing' the therapist in a variety of ways. I recognized a similar process in my work with Jake.

Margot Sunderland (2006: 25–26) uses recent neuroscientific research to explain how physical interactive play produces natural brain chemicals connected with wellbeing, such as opioid hormones and oxytocin. She suggests that 'interactive play can enhance the emotion-regulating functions in the frontal lobes, helping children to manage their feelings better' (2006:

104). This idea confirms Johnson's claim of the power of the playspace to create the conditions to effect change.

As well as allowing me to witness his suffering, the work also provided an opportunity to model in the here and now a positive and safe relationship between a boy and a man. We shared cooperation, respect, trust, humour and fun.

From being a boy with a problem, Jake was able to take on a role of skilled, creative person, for which I regularly complimented him. Within the dramatherapy, Jake was able to develop a complex dramatic language. We each took on characters and improvised. Jake initiated complex role reversals, where he acted me and I acted him, and then Frank became either him or me, or either of us took on the role of Frank. In any case, Frank seemed to be a kind of alter ego for Jake. Jake introduced dramatic devices such as switching a light off and on to denote a change of scene, or a shift from dreamspace to reality. The scenes transformed themselves rapidly. A story with puppets could suddenly turn into role-play, and vice versa. Amidst the sometimes brutal storylines, there were sudden moments of laughter at the absurdity of something. Importantly, humour was never far away.

It is very important for the young person that the dramatherapist is working with the larger pastoral team. Outside of the dramatherapy, Jake received support and nurture from a Pastoral Assistant in the school. I doubt if my weekly interventions would have been sufficient without that. The Deputy Head was extremely supportive of my creative and physical approach to the work.

A comparison with verbal approaches

An interesting question is how would this approach compare with a verbal psychotherapeutic approach? One way to look at it is to consider Jake's dramatic skill and energy, and to remember that this is a boy who, when he is asked a question in real life, looks down, becomes listless, and answers monosyllabically. The life seems to drain out of him. Like many other boys, Jake could not even begin to use words to describe his experiences. A verbally-based approach would, I suggest, not have worked for him. By contrast, in the dramatherapy playspace there is direct eye contact, energy, humour, and flowing dialogue. The use of imagination and projection offered by an arts therapy was helpful to him, and the embodiment, and possibility, of physical contact enabled within dramatherapy was particularly useful.

For someone with Jake's needs, given the failure of previous attempts to engage him in purely verbal, reality-based interactions, a creative play- or arts-based approach is preferable.

Developmental Transformations is an approach that has a lot to offer young people like Jake. I have developed my use of this model in my individual work with young people, and have found that the approach has been effective. It is essential that this work is done by trained professional dramatherapists. Meanwhile, more research on this use of DvT in schools is needed.

Conclusion

As shown, dramatherapists working as Primary Mental Health Workers can offer new opportunities to work effectively with young people within schools. A great advantage of 1:1 dramatherapy for boys with behaviour problems is that even where background information is sketchy and boys are not very verbal, drama presents a rich medium where experiences and feelings can be worked through in a safe way to create deep and lasting changes.

References

Bannister, A. (1993) 'Images and action: Dramatherapy and psychodrama with sexually abused adolescents', in S. Jennings (ed.), *Dramatherapy with Children and Adolescents*. Hove: Routledge.

Bannister, A. (2003) 'The effects of creative therapy with children who have been sexually abused', *Dramatherapy* 25 (1), 3–9.

Biddulph, S. (1997) *Raising Boys*. London: Thorsons.

British Association of Dramatherapists Code of Conduct (2005) www.badth.org.

Brown, D. and Pedder, J. (1979) *Introduction to Psychotherapy: An Outline of Psychodynamic Principles and Practice*. London: Tavistock Publications.

Cattanach, A. (1992a) *Play Therapy with Abused Children*. London: Jessica Kingsley.

Cattanach, A. (1992b) *Play Therapy and Dramatic Play with Young Children Who Have Been Abused*. London: Routledge.

Christensen, J. (2010) 'Making a space inside: The experience of dramatherapy within a school-based student support unit', in V. Karkou (ed.), *Arts Therapies in Schools: Research and Practice*. London: Jessica Kingsley.

Emunah, R. (1995) 'From adolescent trauma to adolescent drama: Group drama with emotionally disturbed youth', in S. Jennings (ed.), *Dramatherapy with Children and Adolescents*. Hove: Routledge.

Health Advisory Service (1995) *Together We Stand*. London: HMSO.

James, M., Forrester, A., and Kim, K. (2005) 'Developmental transformations in the treatment of sexually abused children', in A. Weber and C. Haen (eds.), *Clinical Applications of Drama Therapy in Child and Adolescent Treatment*. New York: Brunner Routledge.

Jennings, S. (1990) *Waiting in the Wings*. London: Jessica Kingsley.

Johnson, D. (1991) 'The theory and technique of transformations in drama therapy', *Arts in Psychotherapy*, 18, 285–300.

Johnson, D., Forrester, A., Dintino, C., James, M., and Schnee, G. (1996) 'Towards a poor dramatherapy', *Arts in Psychotherapy*, 23, 383–396.

Johnstone, K. (1981) *Impro: Improvisation and the Theatre*. London: Methuen.

Kolbo, J.R., Blakely, E.H., and Engleman, D. (1996) 'Children who witness domestic violence: A review of empirical literature', *Journal of Interpersonal Violence*, 11 (2), 281–293.

Landy, R. (1992) 'One-on-one: The role of the dramatherapist working with individuals', in S. Jennings (ed.), *Dramatherapy: Theory and Practice 2*. London: Routledge.

Quibell, T. (2010) 'The searching drama of disaffection: dramatherapy groups in a whole-school context', in V. Karkou (ed.), *Arts Therapies in Schools: Research and Practice*. London: Jessica Kingsley.

Social Policy Research Unit (2004) *The Drivers of Social Exclusion: A review of the literature for the Social Exclusion Unit in the Breaking the Cycle series – Summary*. Wetherby, West Yorkshire: Office of the Deputy Prime Minister.

Sunderland, M. (2006) *The Science of Parenting*. London: DK Publishing.

8 All the better to see you with: healing metaphors in a case of sexual abuse

Ann Dix

Another world

Imagine for a moment that you are walking down a road. On one side there is an old tennis court, nets long gone and broken glass sparkling like diamonds on the crumbling asphalt. On the other side of the road are boarded-up houses, with brown metal grills over the windows. The gardens are overgrown and the rubbish blows in the breeze. However, some houses are still inhabited: the curtains closed against the world, but with signs of family life amongst the emptiness. Litter, old mattresses and broken glass lie everywhere.

This could be the beginning of a guided fantasy, but it is a real place. This area was once one of Europe's biggest council estates, currently undergoing a massive regeneration which will take up to 20 years to complete. Huge swathes of social housing are being demolished, with families moved elsewhere in the city, and there are many boarded-up homes, with the attendant rubbish and squalor. There are currently no play areas and there is a sense of decay. Life is hard and it takes some imagination to create any beauty out of this.

> *Wayne was eight and when asked to imagine a place where he might feel safe, drew a house with four boarded-up windows and a barricaded front door. He was unable to describe a safe place and used the reality around him to express his fears. It may have felt safe for him inside, but it appeared a bleak and hopeless vision.*

This is where the children I work with live. They attend the local schools and, for many, the boundaries of the estate are the edges of their worlds. Poverty of life experience, financial insecurity, poor housing and lack of recreational space is a powerful combination, yet there is a sense of community within this area. The local schools have strong pastoral systems which support both the pupils and their families, working closely with other agencies.

There is a realization that many inner city children and their families have multiple needs that require multi-faceted, practical support.

Therapeutic work is essential to meet the needs of the growing number of children and adolescents at risk of mental health difficulties. Not all families are the same and support needs to be targeted in a way that suits individual needs. However, sometimes this fails to address the real issues of poverty and abuse, as we are bombarded with stories of feral children in the press and on TV that demonize the young and provoke knee-jerk reactions by policy makers. In order to reach these children effectively, 'the primary task is to work systemically and across their range of needs' (Batmanghelidjh 2006, 2009).

The case for therapeutic work

There are increasing numbers of children who find it difficult to cope in school, and whose behaviour is often untenable within a school setting. They may have behavioural problems, be quiet and withdrawn or have experienced loss and separation. These children are a cause for concern to schools, particularly when their behaviour disrupts their opportunities for learning.

All these young people can benefit from therapeutic work, and there are a growing number of creative arts therapists working in schools, using arts therapies to help young people express themselves in a safe and creative way. As Camilleri states 'Creative arts therapies allow children to tap into their creative imaginations and use this resource for connection, growth and healing' (2007: 71), so enabling them to become more resilient and emotionally literate.

I work as a dramatherapist in a multi-agency support team, based within the community. Many families struggle with multiple difficulties, including poverty, disability and mental illness, as well as fear of violence and abuse. Most parents lack parenting skills, have had little experience of a positive upbringing themselves, and struggle to provide boundaries for their children, but want the best for them. Dramatherapy is offered in order to encourage the child to find alternative ways of behaving, and think differently about their lives.

Dramatherapy and creativity

Dramatherapy is defined as the 'intentional use of the healing aspects of drama and theatre as the therapeutic process' and a way of working that 'uses action methods to facilitate creativity, imagination, learning, insight and growth' (British Association of Dramatherapists mission statement; badth.org.uk). There are several models of dramatherapy, but I find the Creative Expressive method as developed by Sue Jennings (1990) and outlined in McFarlane (2005: 5) to be the most useful and child friendly. The use of embodiment–projection–role allows children to replicate the stages of child development and revisit those stages they may have missed.

It is sometimes difficult to imagine how children can be creative when they exist in a world of boarded-up houses, or they have been badly abused, and yet repeatedly they use stories and create images to express their thoughts and tell of their distress. Sometimes these stories are too painful to speak about, but through the use of metaphor they can be enacted and thought about, in order to find some kind of resolution. This allows for a 'degree of "aesthetic distance"' (Jennings 1990; Landy 1993: 25) so that the child is not emotionally flooded and can maintain a sense of control through the manipulation of symbolic arts materials (Miller et al. 2005). These stories can help to engender a sense of hope for the future.

Dramatherapy is a powerful method of addressing children's needs and the following case study demonstrates how Claire uses fairy stories as a metaphor for some events in her life. The therapy took place in school, where she was supported by teachers and a learning mentor.

Initial assessment

Claire was 11, lived with foster carers and attended a local school. She had a younger brother, Joe, who was adopted elsewhere, and with whom she had no contact. Claire wanted to see Joe and her social worker was trying to organize this. She talked a lot about her hopes for this meeting. Claire's mother was dead, and Claire had been sexually abused at the age of 6 by a teenage family friend. Claire appeared friendly and outgoing, and was very anxious that I should like her. I had been told by her carer that she stole, frequently told lies at school and home, and was very destructive of her possessions, but Claire was keen for me to know that she didn't always do this. She was able to talk openly about her abuse, and the death of her mother shortly before she was received into care, but appeared split between the unemotional way she told her life story and the extreme behaviours she sometimes exhibited. 'Sexually abused children frequently present as emotionally distant, distrustful, aggressive and hyper-vigilant due to their expectations of being abused by others' (Miller et al. 2005: 71). Claire was unable to accept praise and would react by breaking something or having a major tantrum shortly afterwards. She was unable to keep things she liked and would destroy her toys and books.

I had several multi-agency meetings with her learning mentor, foster carer and social worker before finally meeting Claire. Looked-after children may require specialist intervention because of long-term attachment issues (Archer and Burnell 2003). It is important to have an understanding of the child's history in order to put behaviours into context; however, it is also important to have an open mind when meeting the child, so as not to allow the opinions of others to influence one's own impressions.

Clearly, Claire found it difficult to make a close bond with anyone, although on first meeting she appeared overly friendly and obliging. She spent her first few sessions testing me out. Her disorganized form of attachment is common in children who have been fostered or adopted (Bowlby 1969; Main and Hesse 1990; Archer and Burnell 2003).

Engaging with the metaphor

We began work using tactile materials to encourage Claire to use physical movement in a non-threatening way (embodiment), which led to the projection of ideas onto an object.

> *In our early sessions we created a butterfly out of papier mache, which she painted in jewel colours. I thought it was interesting that she would choose this image and we talked about the journey from caterpillar to butterfly. I had a sense that Claire was trying to emerge from her cocoon, but felt trapped inside herself. The butterfly was finished with silver wings. Claire was able to project her unspoken feelings onto this image and the physical manipulation of the materials encouraged her to talk about her abuse and her longing to see her brother again. She also talked about her feelings towards other members of her family, and how she felt they had not protected her. In particular, she spoke about her Gran, who she felt had ignored her when she had tried to disclose the abuse.*
>
> *This was played out in a later session, when Claire chose puppets to act out a meeting between herself and Joe. In her story, Claire told of a real visit she had made to see Joe and Gran, who made tea for them. The Claire puppet was able to hold Joe puppet and nurse him, while Gran puppet nurtured her with food and drink. I asked her what she would like to have happened and she moved the puppets so that Gran was holding Claire and Joe and telling them she loved them both. Claire made Gran say 'I won't let you go. I love you both.'*

Claire used both sensory embodiment and projection to create and give voice to her story. She worked with metaphor in creating the butterfly, but developed the story through 'dramatic play' (Jennings 1990: 15). Claire took factual events but recreated the scene she wished for, allowing herself autonomy by reconstructing the story so that she had more power. Through the puppet voice she was able to hear the 'I love you' that she had not experienced in reality.

> *We did not return to story making for several weeks after this. Claire chose to play games that had clear rules and boundaries, and continued to test me out with questions and lies, after which she was always anxious to check that I still liked her and wasn't angry. We talked about her anger and her ambivalent feelings towards people, but she found it very difficult to express her emotions authentically. She often disowned feelings that seemed unacceptable or threatening to her sense of self (Perl 2008: 141). She continued to present herself as a cheerful, smiling girl, and gave little*

away of the sadness and anger inside her. I was reminded of Winnicott's description of the compliant false self, masking the true self (Winnicott 1971: 102). It was several months into our work when Claire announced that she liked me because I told her the truth and I realized that she had stopped trying to catch me out by challenging everything I said.

The role of the therapist in school

Claire was beginning to appear more settled in school, and was getting good reports, which was having a positive effect on her foster placement. It appeared that Claire was beginning to use her creativity to process her past and contemplate her future. I had many discussions with her learning mentor, in order to put the work into context. This meant holding Claire's confidentiality but also giving pointers to school as to the reasons for some of her behaviours.

It is important not to mystify the process of therapy, but to try to be as clear and open as possible, in order to encourage schools to feel confident about having therapists on the premises. It is also important for the therapist to maintain a consistent presence for the child. This includes trying to see the child in the same place and at the same time each week. When working in schools, this is not always possible, as school trips, exams and other activities take precedence, but it is my experience that children are flexible enough to understand that they might move session times or work on a different day. When I have asked the children I work with what they would prefer, they usually say that they want to come at a different time rather than miss a session, which leads me to think that the therapeutic alliance between therapist and client provides a strong enough boundary for this to work. However, consistency and boundary-holding is particularly important for children who may not experience it elsewhere in their lives.

Choosing a role and creating a drama

In session 16 Claire asked if we could use the digital camera in session, and I explained that as part of our Child Protection policy, we would print any picture for her to keep, but that we would delete them from the camera at the end of the session. Prior agreement with her carer and school had been obtained. Once in the playroom, Claire found the dressing up clothes she wanted for her story. She had chosen Little Red Riding Hood.

Little Red Riding Hood is a tale of the loss of childhood innocence and is sometimes associated with sexual abuse. Bettlelheim describes fairy stories as speaking to 'our conscious and our unconscious' (1975: 174) and there are obvious parallels for Claire; Grandma is not able to protect Claire from the wolf, who is able to come into the house and take control. Claire's confusion about sex and her sometimes inappropriate sexual behaviours can be seen in the context of the charming but manipulative behaviour of the wolf.

> *Claire decided she would be Red Riding Hood and I could be Mum, the Wolf, Grandma and the Woodcutter. We dressed up in the pieces of material in the room and began the story, with Claire directing the action. When we got to the part where the wolf was going to eat Red Riding Hood, Claire screamed and ran away, saying she didn't want to be eaten. We decided to repeat this section again so that she could experience the power of saying 'No', and in Claire's version of the story, Red Riding Hood was not eaten. The woodcutter appears and kills the Wolf and rescues Grandma. Claire decided that she wanted photographs of herself as Red Riding Hood and me as the Wolf and Grandma. Then she moved to a different area of the room and found the big baby doll, which she gave to me. She took a photograph of me, in the role of Grandma, holding the baby doll and then a second photo of me, as the therapist, holding the carrycot with the baby doll inside.*

In this session, Claire had moved into role play, thus completing the embodiment–projection–role paradigm, although she continued to move freely between all three. As Jennings says, the dramatic imagination is crucial for survival and a key factor in adolescent maturation (Jennings 1990, 1995). Claire was able to take control of the story, change it, replay it and create the symbolic photographs of the events she emotionally craved. By having actual photographs she was able to concretize her feelings whilst being able to differentiate between fantasy and reality.

It was important for her to have the power to say 'no' to the wolf, and to not be eaten (or abused) and also to explore the relationship with Grandma, who, in reality, had been unable to keep her safe, but who in the story was rescued and then photographed holding a baby. The two photographs of me, as Grandma and as myself, holding the baby seem to represent Claire's need for her inner child to be protected, whilst also challenging my ability as therapist to keep her safe. Claire struggled with attachments, but appeared able to project her desires onto myself and the doll.

This role-play clearly demonstrated the therapeutic performance process (need identifying, rehearsal, showing and disengagement) outlined in Jones (1996: 102), allowing Claire to create her story and change her relationship to the material during the dramatization.

> *In the following sessions we enacted Cinderella and Snow White. Claire was able to direct the action and role reverse. The themes of 'good and bad mother' figured in each. In both stories, the birth mother is dead and we paused and replayed the moment of death, taking a photo to capture*

the moment. At one point, Cinderella (Claire) shouted out 'my mother is dead' and the pain in her voice was chilling. She explored the death of Snow White by creating a coffin of cushions and decorating it with flowers, and again we took a photograph of her lying in state, before moving on to the awakening. Both stories finished with Claire, dressed as a bride, looking beautiful and marrying the Prince.

Claire explored death and grief by replaying these scenes until they became more bearable. Using metaphor gave her a sense of safety through aesthetic distance so that she could say 'this is me' and 'this is not me'. 'The dramatic distancing in itself provides a structure for participants that paradoxically bring them closer to themselves' (Jennings 1990: 210).

The following session recapped all the roles we had played, and we took more photographs of the characters, allowing Claire to revisit and re-experience the key moments in her drama.

Evaluation

At the end of this piece of work we reviewed our sessions and talked about our work together. We created a scrapbook of the photographs and wrote comments about the scenes they represented as a permanent record. The pictures showed Claire expressing a number of emotions, including sadness and anger, and she was able to acknowledge this. Claire wrote her own words under each picture describing the scenes. She was extremely proud of her book and took it away with her to show her teacher. Her self evaluation said 'Nobody thinks I could do this. I'm good'.

It seemed as though Claire became less self-critical as she found 'that another person can accept and even enjoy parts of herself that she has rejected' (Perl 2008: 42). This helped Claire to begin to tolerate those aspects of herself that she did not like or want to accept. As Perl goes on to say: 'When others encounter parts of her personality that might actually be difficult or unappealing but sustain their love or regard, they might help her to hold onto different . . . conflicting feelings about herself' (2008: 42).

Claire had formed a positive attachment with me, but still found it difficult to acknowledge her feelings of trust and affection, although it was important for her to know that I liked and trusted her.

Claire's learning mentor and social worker confirmed that her behaviour was calmer at school and home, and she was achieving better grades academically. Also she appeared to be getting on better with her peers, and there were fewer angry outbursts. Her carer said that Claire was more able to talk to her and that the stealing had lessened. She had also noticed that Claire would sometimes hug her spontaneously.

Dramatherapy in schools can be a most effective way of reaching traumatized young people. It can bridge a gap between disaffected youth and the school, and enable young people to feel listened to and held safely.

The therapist is seen as a neutral figure who can support the child in addressing their social and emotional needs, and bring added value to a busy school. The therapist is also able to listen to the child's story, particularly when it contains painful events that the child does not want to talk about to teachers who are also responsible for their discipline and education. As the case study illustrates, the use of symbolic play and role-play can be especially effective in allowing the child to practice new ways of thinking and behaving in a creative and sustainable way.

References

Archer, C. and Burnell, A. (2003) *Trauma, Attachment and Family Permanence. Fear Can Stop You Loving*. London: Jessica Kingsley.

Batmanghelidjh, C. (2006) *Shattered Lives. Children who live with courage and dignity*. London: Jessica Kingsley.

Batmanghelidjh, C. (2009) 'Terrorised and terrorising teenagers: the search for attachment and hope', in A. Perry (ed.), *Teenagers and Attachment. Helping Adolescents Engage with Life and Learning*. London: Worth.

Bettlelheim, B. (1975) *The Uses of Enchantment. The Meaning and Importance of Fairy Tale*. London: Penguin.

Bowlby, J. (1969) *Attachment and Loss. Volume 1*. London: Hogarth Press.

Camilleri, V.A. (ed.) (2007) *Healing the Inner City Child. Creative Arts Therapies with At-Risk Youth*. London: Jessica Kingsley.

Jennings, S. (1990) *Dramatherapy with Families, Groups and Individuals. Waiting in the Wings*. London: Jessica Kingsley.

Jennings, S. (ed.) (1995) *Dramatherapy with Children and Adolescents*. London: Routledge.

Jones, P. (1996) *Drama as Therapy. Theatre as Living*. London: Routledge.

Landy, R. (1993) *Persona and Performance. The Meaning of Role in Dramatherapy and Everyday Life*. London: Jessica Kingsley.

Main, M. and Hesse, E. (1990) 'The insecure disorganised/disorientated attachment pattern in infancy: Precursors and sequelae', in M. Greenberg, D. Cicchetti, and E.M. Cummings (eds.), *Attachment During the Preschool Years. Theory, Research and Intervention*. Chicago: University of Chicago Press.

McFarlane, P. (2005) *Dramatherapy. Developing Emotional Stability*. London: David Fulton.

Miller, J., Forrester, A.M., and Kim, K.C. (2005) 'Developmental transformations in the treatment of sexually abused children', in A.M. Weber and C. Haen (eds.), *Clinical Applications of Drama Therapy in Child and Adolescent Treatment*. East Sussex: Brunner-Routledge.

Perl, E. (2008) *Psychotherapy with Adolescent Girls and Young Women. Fostering Autonomy Through Attachment*. New York: Guildford Press.

Winnicott, D.W. (1971) *Playing and Reality*. London: Routledge.

9 *Romeo and Juliet* and dramatic distancing: chaos and anger contained for inner-city adolescents in multicultural schools

Mandy Carr

Introduction: image as the language of adolescence

Adolescence can be viewed as a time of transition from child to adulthood, where a cocktail of hormones and changes to body and mind can create anger and confusion. Although this may seem a modern problem, teenagers through the ages in different ways have shared the same fears and difficulties. In this chapter I intend to examine how *Romeo and Juliet*, Shakespeare's play about teenage love and family tensions, may be used in dramatherapy sessions to help reflect issues in the twenty-first century. I will examine how Shakespeare reaches out to troubled young people whose unexpressed anger may be impeding their educational and emotional development.

Karkou (2010: 13) notes that children at risk of developing mental health problems can have their initial contact with qualified professionals in school. Difficulties can thus be identified and addressed early, without resorting to specialized services outside the school environment. This chapter aims to show the impact of the work on the resilience of young people from a variety of cultures as well as the importance of providing therapeutic interventions within a school context.

Two case studies are used to demonstrate how issues in the play *Romeo and Juliet* can support teenagers in expressing and processing their anger in a therapeutic context, enabling them to develop the coping skills and emotional resilience to function and fulfil their educational potential. The first case study will explore the use of parental themes from *Romeo and Juliet* with an adolescent boy on the autistic spectrum, in a special school. The second will describe a story devised by a 12-year-old girl to process bullying issues in an inner-city secondary school, following her engagement with the theme of tension between the Montagues and Capulets. Whilst these cases are fictitious, they are based on an amalgam of young people's experiences within dramatherapy. Teenagers often find it difficult to talk about their feelings. Dramatherapy provides a confidential space in which young people can discover a sense of safety and freedom to explore their emotions and inner world through creative arts work. If we ask an adolescent how they are, they will probably say 'OK'. Ask them to express how they are through movement, an image or a sound, and a different story and sense of release will emerge. 'If you want to speak to troubled children or have them speak to you, you are far more likely to be successful if you do it through their language – the language of image, metaphor or story' (Frankel 1998: 108).

Romeo and Juliet: unspeakable adolescent rage with the world

Alida Gersie has written widely on the potential therapeutic benefits of confronting emotionally upsetting events in story form. She notes that the telling of stories 'safeguards our capacity to live through dark nights of the soul. It enables both teller and listener to negotiate fears, to strengthen resolve' (Gersie 1997: 15).

This case study focuses on how the story of *Romeo and Juliet* was utilized within dramatherapy sessions to support a child who was experiencing emotional abuse by a parent. This was done by enabling him to begin to explore his fear, anxiety and suppressed rage. The inner-city special school that he attended caters for young people with moderate learning difficulties.

Aleksander was a 14-year-old boy from an Eastern European background, with a diagnosis of autism. He found it difficult to identify or articulate emotions and to empathize with others, and did not show interest in communicating with his peers. He was, however, imaginative and loved performing. Furthermore, his cognitive language skills were good, and only slightly below average for his age. In the classroom he had become increasingly anxious and withdrawn. Each lesson started with a circle time of six to eight students and Aleksander had become unable to join the group. When he tried, he would sit trembling, rocking backwards and forwards, moaning or talking to himself. Eventually he was withdrawn from the classroom to work in a quiet room with a support assistant. One could argue that his desire to withdraw was further compounded by his anxiety.

Cattanach quotes Kanner's 1943 description of autism, cited by Wing (1976) as 'a profound withdrawal from contact with people, an obsessive desire for the preservation of sameness . . . the kind of language that does not seem intended to serve inter-personal communication' (Cattanach 1996: 86).

Aleksander's home situation was complex. His father found the challenge of a teenage boy with autism difficult and had become autocratic in his response to the boy, allowing him no freedom, frequently locking him in his bedroom for hours at a time. Concerns were raised with Social Care and Aleksander was placed on the Child Protection Register. This caused a breakdown in communication between the school and Aleksander's parents, who became angry and distrustful. As a consequence of this, Aleksander's levels of anxiety became heightened.

Aleksander was terrified of his father, who had forbidden him from speaking about his home life at school. Aleksander was studying *Romeo and Juliet* and in his dramatherapy sessions he chose to focus on the scene in which Juliet's father hits and insults her, because she will not marry Parris. Talking of his daughter, Capulet comments:

> 'I think she will be ruled in all respects by me.'
> (Shakespeare 2004. *Romeo and Juliet* Act 3, Scene 4: 13)

Juliet begs her father to listen to her:

> 'Good father. I beseech you on my knees, Hear me with patience but to speak a word.'
> (Shakespeare 2004. *Romeo and Juliet* Act 3, Scene 5: 160)

Initially Aleksander chose to work with the character of Juliet. He directed the dramatherapist to stand and represent Juliet, then took on Juliet's position himself, delivering her line, 'Good father. . .'. He experimented with different ways of standing, moving and speaking, then he repeated the process with the role of father. Aleksander began to develop the scenes, improvising his own lines, and trying out different strategies, to persuade Juliet's 'father' to see her point of view.

He discussed the feelings of both characters with the dramatherapist and took on the role of an observer, commenting on the 'bullying' behaviour of the father and the victimization of his daughter. He experimented with different postures for the roles of the father and of Juliet to experience the different feelings of power and control. Eventually, he created a movement piece in which he started with the 'victim' posture he had created for Juliet (kneeling, head bowed) and he transformed slowly to the 'bully' posture of the father (standing, hand raised ready to hit). Aleksander located a posture that he felt most comfortable with, standing feet firmly on the ground, his arms reaching out, apparently ready to communicate. In this 'affirming' posture, he commented as an observer that Juliet had been treated unfairly, should be allowed to make her own decisions and should never be hit. He explored the breathing patterns, physicality, posture and quality of voice elicited, and experimented with how he could use this in his own life to overcome anxiety.

Chesner (1995) views the use of role within dramatherapy as a significant factor in empowering people with learning disabilities. She discusses how established patterns of behaviour can be overcome through experimenting with posture, breathing, facial expression and thought patterns. 'Dramatherapy is helpful in encouraging people to expand their role repertoire . . . People with learning disabilities, whose role repertoires tend to be limited, can discover other modes of expression and new possibilities in their own lives through playing with role in the context of dramatherapy' (Chesner 1995: 7).

Aleksander was not asked to comment on the details of his own life situation, and his anxiety was the only aspect of his personal life mentioned. All other feelings and dilemmas were discussed over six weekly sessions within the metaphor of the piece of drama he had chosen.

Teachers noticed that during this period he was able to join his classes and contain his anxiety. With the staff I shared strategies that I considered successful, through pastoral referral meetings. Strategies, which included the use of breathing exercises and self talk, were with Aleksander's permission shared with parents and staff, and incorporated into his individual education plan and utilized when appropriate. Aleksander appeared to be happy with this outcome, and he requested further dramatherapy sessions.

Storymaking: the transformational potential of developing broader perspectives

Gabriela was an 11-year-old girl attending an inner-city comprehensive school that had a significant number of refugees, with 59 different languages. It was situated in an area of extreme social deprivation. The school was aware of the need for therapeutic work with many of its students and a separate building housed counselling, dramatherapy and musictherapy.

Gabriela and her family had come from Columbia when she was nine years old. It was believed the family had left the country because of increasing violence, but little was known of her background. Gabriella did not speak fluent English, which added to her frustrations in making herself understood. She had been referred because she had been fighting and verbally abusing staff. She seemed visibly relieved when offered the chance to see if dramatherapy might be helpful.

In my experience, young people regularly make comments like, 'I've had counselling, but how can I talk about this stuff?' Dramatherapy allows them to choose which issues to work with through creative methods, rather than discussion. The work began to engage Gabriela by using techniques developed by the Brazilian director Augusto Boal (1992). One of Gabriela's initial activities was to participate in a structure known as 'Image Dialogue', where dramatherapist and client start by creating together a non-verbal image of two people shaking hands. The client steps out, while the therapist remains frozen in the image. The client examines the image of the therapist with hand outstretched, and joins her to create a new image. The therapist then steps out and creates another image, and so it goes on. Thus a spontaneous dialogue/dance is created wholly through movement. Gabriela's images demonstrated a polarity between connection and closeness, antagonism and distance. At the end of this activity, she reflected on the images she had created and decided that they represented friendship, fighting and rejection.

She went on to explore the themes of friendship and fighting, using Act 1 Scene 1 of *Romeo and Juliet* as a stimulus. This is the scene in which

Samson and Gregory, Capulet servants, taunt and fight with Abraham, a Montague. The lines are accessible and easy for young people, even those who are new to English, to express through voice and movement:

Abraham: Do you bite your thumb at us, sir?
Samson: I do bite my thumb, sir.
Abraham: Do you bite your thumb at us, sir?
Samson: No, sir, I do not bite my thumb at you, sir, but I bite my thumb, sir.

(Shakespeare 2004. *Romeo and Juliet* Act 1, Scene 1: 43–49)

Gabriela had told me that a common classroom experience was that girls would call her names, for example, 'Freshie', referring to her as a newcomer to the UK. She would then get angry, start a fight, then be blamed by the teacher, who she would tell to 'F. . . off'. She had a profound sense of injustice, but was prevented from explaining her perspective to the teacher, partly by her overwhelming anger, also by her lack of fluency in English. She played the above scene, alternating both roles with the therapist, who directed the movement and tone of voice. The final time she played the scene, her anger turned to tears. She cried for about ten minutes, witnessed and supported by the dramatherapist.

In the next session, Gabriela played the role of a mediator between Samson and Abraham. In that role, she insisted that Abraham apologize to Samson for taunting him in the first place. She was invited to reflect on which strategies might help her in the classroom. Gabriela wanted to be able to explain her situation to adults when things went wrong for her. She agreed to take part in 'restorative justice' meetings, a peer mediation system run by the school. She expressed interest in training to become a peer mediator herself. These strategies were passed on to the school and family.

The experience of dramatherapy provided Gabriela with therapeutic 'tools' to develop the resilience she needed within school and her home life. Working with themes that she had identified through movement rather than discussion, as well as the dramatic distance created by *Romeo and Juliet*, enabled her to reflect upon difficult issues. She was able to develop a vocabulary to articulate her feelings, rather than acting them out inappropriately. Given that she was not yet fluent in English, this was crucially important. Renee Emunah describes the process whereby a teenager can learn more controlled ways of expressing potentially overwhelming feelings by giving them expression within the safe boundaries of character and story: 'Rather than complete immersion in the rage, in which nothing else but feeling exists, the actor is aware of him or herself. Strong feeling is not suppressed but mastered' (Emunah 1995: 154). Furthermore, Gabriela had created a trusting relationship with the therapist through a variety of creative conversations.

Evaluations by young clients and their teachers

Thirty-two young people who had worked with dramatherapy in the two schools, including those mentioned in the case studies, were invited to complete a questionnaire, in which they were given a series of statements to tick and to add their own comments about their experiences. Their ticks showed:

> 100% said that they enjoyed acting out stories
> 90% said it helped them to understand other people and communicate more clearly
> 80% said that they felt 'listened to'
> 70% said that it helped them to manage their behaviour
> 40% said that it helped them to feel good about themselves.

Comments included 'When we're angry we can move the anger away from us and control it', and 'I had fun and let out my feelings'.

Their form tutors were also asked to evaluate the impact of dramatherapy on their pupils and school life:

> 80% noticed a slight or noticeable improvement in listening skills and empathy and social skills
> 60% saw a noticeable improvement in working with others
> 40% noticed a significant improvement in behaviour management.

It has been widely reported that many teachers find the behaviour of young people challenging. Seven out of ten teachers responding to a survey in Teachers' TV 'cited pupils' behaviour among the most stressful aspects of the job' (Carr and Ramsden 2009: 183). It is significant therefore that teachers in this project responded positively to dramatherapy as an intervention that supported young people in learning to manage their behaviour.

Conclusion: dramatherapy as container for adolescent tensions

Dramatherapy can afford adolescents the opportunity to find healthy ways of expressing chaos or anger, and it offers them opportunities to develop coping mechanisms and emotional resilience. Jennings notes how Shakespeare's plays can create opportunities to make profound psychological shifts, regardless of linguistic or cultural background. 'The characters, themselves, give us insight into human nature, and the very language transports us into realms of communication we could not otherwise achieve' (1992, 16).

Jennings cites Cox's seminal work (1988), which demonstrates how primordial communication from people with no knowledge of Shakespeare can be expressed through metaphors that can help facilitate intrapsychic change. The two case studies in this chapter blend the clients' connection with Shakespearian themes of parental authority, friendship, bullying and emerging adolescent identity with the creation of a trusting, authentic relationship with the dramatherapist. Moreover, the links between the therapist, school and home are crucial in supporting the young person's development, as well as the opportunity to work through creative media.

'Caught between the pulls of dependency and responsibility, no longer a child, but not yet an adult, the adolescent bears the tension of the opposites in a dramatic way' (Frankel 1998: 5). The therapeutic use of Shakespearian themes can support young people in learning to bear the tension, to express chaos and anger in a safe place and, through this, to start to develop the coping mechanisms necessary to survive and thrive in an educational setting and in their broader lives.

References

Boal, A. (1992) *Games for Actors and Non-Actors*. London: Routledge.

Carr, M. and Ramsden, E. (2009) 'An exploration of supervision in education', in D. Dokter and P. Jones (eds.), *Supervision of Dramatherapy*. London: Routledge.

Cattanach, A. (1996) *Drama for People with Special Needs*. London: A & C Black.

Chesner, A. (1995) *Dramatherapy for People with Learning Disabilities: A World of Difference*. London: Jessica Kingsley.

Emunah, R. (1995) 'From adolescent trauma to adolescent drama: Group drama therapy with emotionally disturbed youth', in S. Jennings (ed.), *Dramatherapy with Children and Adolescents*, London: Routledge.

Frankel, R. (1998) *The Adolescent Psyche: Jungian and Winnicottian Perspectives*. New York: Brunner-Routledge.

Gersie, A. (1997) *Reflections on Therapeutic Storymaking: The Use of Stories in Groups*. London: Jessica Kingsley.

Jennings, S. (1992) 'Therapeutic journeys through *King Lear*', in S. Jennings (ed.), *Dramatherapy: Theory and Practice 2*. London: Routledge.

Karkou, K. (2010) *Arts Therapies in Schools, Research and Practice*. London: Jessica Kingsley.

Shakespeare, W. (2004) *Romeo and Juliet*. New York: Washington Square Press.

Wing, L. (1976) 'Problems of diagnosis and classification', in L. Everard (ed.), *An Approach to Teaching Autistic Children*. Oxford: Pergamon.

10 Looking for meaning with bereaved children and families: 'Bring back my Daddy' and other stories

Roya Dooman

It is not always obvious who may be the first person in school to notice a child's or family's distress. In the case of bereavement it may well be the family themselves who ask for support because 1 in 29 school-aged children have experienced the death of a parent or sibling (Fauth et al. 2009). Bereavement can lead to extreme stress, putting huge demands on a family's ability to cope. As professionals, if we ignore the impact of profound grief on family life, we are ignoring research that links unresolved grief in childhood with adult depression and mental ill health. The childhood bereavement network (www.childhoodbereavementnetwork.org.uk) states that 55% of bereaved children are more likely to have a diagnosable mental health disorder, and the research of Abdelnoor and Hollins (2004) demonstrates 60% of children who have lost a parent or sibling are more likely to be excluded from school and may underachieve at GCSE (Fauth et al. 2009). Jewett confirms 'Growing evidence links childhood loss with depression, alcoholism, anxiety, and suicidal tendencies in adolescence and adulthood' (1997: vi).

Profound grief can feel as if the roots of a family have been cruelly ripped out, leaving it vulnerable and disconnected. An important relationship has been lost and belief systems are threatened, affecting all established and new relationships. Engaging in everyday life with all its complexities, such as returning to school after a bereavement, can feel overwhelming. The separate therapy space can offer anchorage to the child and their family, and act as a bridge between understanding their loss and what it means, and the demands of school life. Here, the child can find a place to mourn what is lost and to express her fears about the possibility of it happening again. Gersie's work *Storymaking in Bereavement* (1996) demonstrates that helping people recreate rituals and stories can bring back meaning into their lives. Western theories on bereavement have been dominated by the universal application of 'stages' or tasks of grieving (Fredman 1997: xix). Merely accepting such a thing as 'closure' for the bereaved, so they can leave behind this special relationship and move on, does not allow for a relationship with the deceased in the present nor, importantly, in the future (Silverman and Klass 1996). Bauchsbaum examines how memories of the dead parent can 'act as a bridge between the world with and the world without the loved person' (1996: 113).

Each loss is unique and has its own complexities, therefore we must listen carefully to how and what families tell us about their own particular story (Fredman 1997). In the initial sessions the therapist must find out the background to the death and its context: when and where did the death occur and were any of the family present at the time? Whether the death was sudden or expected after a long illness; if it followed another death, or if the deceased took their own life. It is important to acknowledge the family's coping mechanisms and look at the implications for their future.

We need to ask questions about their cultural beliefs to help explore how death is experienced by members of this family and how their religious and spiritual beliefs affect their current experience of loss. We need to help families find their own resources as to where they will access meaning about death and mortality and how these views may differ from each other (Fredman 1997: 61). A family's personal style of coping and temperament will affect their grief. Coping strategies will also be affected by attachment patterns in their relationships, for when a parent or principal care giver has died, the child's journey through the grief process will be affected by the nature of 'good enough' relationship with the deceased and also with the remaining parent (Bowlby 1980).

Enabling children to find ways to access memories through creative exploration and transform them into new stories can create new symbols of hope for the continuity of that relationship. The dramatherapist can help the family see how their own support network can be strengthened by the school's, often by inviting a family to create a small world 'Sculpt' using objects and small figures to represent family, friends, GP, teachers and staff.

Through the following vignettes I intend to demonstrate how dramatherapy can help to forge a positive relationship with the deceased, which will have a positive effect on the relationships with the living.

Bring back my Daddy

'Within dramatherapy, play processes are part of a deliberate therapeutic programme for working with the client' (Jones 2007: 168). Young children use the dramatherapy sessions to fulfil their needs as long as 'permission to play' is demonstrated by the therapist. The dramatherapist creates the 'safe' place for the child and, within that, the dramatherapist's role is not to interpret but to 'act' within the unfolding drama, only using the 'role' given to him within the child's story (Cattanach 1994: 60–61).

Stephen, a bright six-year-old whose father had died from a painful lung disease, repeatedly tried to resuscitate 'Action Man' on the story mat.

Stephen moved over to the sand tray where he buried Action Man each week, instructing me to bring the other dolls and animals from the mat to mourn him. Each time Stephen chose whether or not he would resurrect the Action Man, testing his own powers of life over death. He knew that 'real' death meant Daddy was never coming back, but in his own drama he led the script.

Stephen had cognitively grasped an understanding of the irreversibility of death as we would expect and yet emotionally, like many adults, was unable to accept its finality and railed against the shock of it happening. His only previous experience of death had been the death of his pet mouse. As Bauchbaum points out 'mourning must be defined in terms of a child's affective, defensive, and cognitive capacities' (1996: 115).

A quiet boy, well behaved at school and home, Stephen had internalized a strong sense of societal 'rules', which he demonstrated in the classroom and that could only be bypassed in the therapy session once he had entered the 'drama' via the play with the puppets.

Stephen used large puppets to express the wild feelings raging inside him as their 'naughtiness' allowed them to do the unthinkable. They 'blew up' parts of the hospital again and again and the explosions caused 'damage and injuries' to the other toys so they too had to go to hospital! Stephen laughed at the chaos this caused. The 'Doctors' , Stephen and the therapist, reinstated normality, at Stephen's request, by asserting the rules and putting order back into the hospital.

Death challenges what we think we know in a rude and frightening manner. Daddy's death had challenged Stephen's view of nurses and doctors as people who make things better and do not let people die; they had broken the rules. In the dramatherapy, Stephen could play out the conflict of these two thoughts.

When Stephen's mother joined Stephen in the sessions we talked about what the 'naughty' puppets were doing in the hospital. Using the language of play, Stephen's mother observed his struggle from an emotional distance and reflected that Stephen had not been permitted to have the information she had received from the doctors about her husband's illness being terminal. She wondered if it might have been helpful for him to have been more prepared for the death.

This drama was repeated over the sessions with different emphases as Stephen's feelings at the injustice of Daddy's death worked their way to consciousness.

Stephen expressed how 'it wasn't fair' that other children still had their daddies and he didn't have his. With Stephen's mother, we began to imagine places where Daddy might be now that he had died. His mother did not hold any religious beliefs in heaven or the afterlife but talked about planting a tree for her husband. Stephen wanted to find a place for Daddy now, so he chose to make a big shiny star and described how they shone at night. Stephen believed if he could whisper to the star, Daddy would hear.

Stephen needed to bring the 'wishful' part of his relationship with his Daddy into the present, so we began recreating visual images from his memory that he could take into his future. 'The availability of early parental memories may permit an essential form of psychic survival, providing the continuity required for the coherent development of the sense of self' (Bauchsbaum 1996: 115).

In the sessions the puppets could now join Stephen creating pictures of him and Daddy 'in the park' or 'on holiday', adding speech bubbles to add an imagined or wished-for dialogue, but always, when 'the missing' became too painful, one of the puppets would create new stunts to 'amaze' the therapist and bring back the right 'aesthetic distance' into the room. 'At aesthetic distance, the individual is capable of feeling, without fear of being overwhelmed by the emotion, and thinking without fear of losing the ability to respond passionately' (Landy 1996: 87).

Gradually the emotional intensity and the pace of the sessions changed and Stephen began to show more resilience in the classroom and the playground and was able to create an ending with the toys and the therapist.

A child's attempt to hold onto a relationship with a dead parent will become challenged over time, as beliefs and meanings around the loss change with life experience. The school may notice this through a significant dip in a child's levels of achievement, academically, as well as socially and emotionally. The dramatherapist can offer groups of children at a later stage in their development opportunities to engage with that enduring relationship through story, which can improve the child's capacity to function in school. Gersie says 'Whether there is ease or dis-ease in our relationship with our dead parent, what often continues to hurt us, years after their death, is that our maturation results in a changing relationship with our parent's deeds and misdeeds' (Gersie 1996: 133). Gersie invites people to work with stories, that will engage the past, present and future in a dynamic relationship with the deceased, extending their bond of attachment.

Two years on from Stephen's initial therapy he was invited to a dramatherapy bereavement group. It was important to ensure that developmentally the group was ready for this shared task using 'role' ('Pre-role check list', Jones 2007: 214) to enable new rituals to be created through the story.

The group constructed new stories from *The Odyssey*, where 'demons' were fought and words were said in a new shared reality through 'role'. In role as Odysseus, Stephen made a picture of 'two tigers' to send back to his son, and the group witnessed Telemachus' astonishment that his father would remember him from 'so far away'.

Stephen could now make connections out of 'role' with another child that both their fathers had died from painful illnesses but were now free of pain: a mature concept that Stephen aged eight could now affectively and cognitively engage with. His relationship with his father was changing but enduring. This would support Silverman and Nickman's analysis of data that showed that children were 'maintaining relationships to their dead parents rather than letting go' (1996: 73). Sadness would always be a feature of their lives, but would not be as debilitating.

Chocolate heaven

Judy was called in to speak to the teacher about her son Chris' difficult behaviour in a Year 2 class. Judy said that she also found him difficult and 'irrationally angry' at home. She believed it was connected to her mother dying earlier in the year and asked for a referral to be made to the dramatherapist for Chris and her elder daughter Sandy in Year 6.

In the first session alone with the children, Chris and Sandy told me they couldn't talk to Mummy about Grandma in case they made her feel 'too sad' and her face became 'all wet again'. Chris said he felt 'cross' with his teachers and 'fed up' with his friends because 'my feelings are muddled up in my tummy'.

Using the puppets on the story mat to act out different feelings around losing Grandma gave Chris an opportunity to see how sad feelings get mixed up with angry ones. Slowly, through play with 'Grumpy Mr Fox', 'Sad Monkey' and the other puppets, Chris began to unravel these feelings for himself.

I guided conversations with his older sister through the puppets, encouraging her to express her feelings, which helped Chris understand for the first time that some of the difficulties around losing someone we love weren't his alone. Projecting feelings onto the puppets could show Chris how everyone in a family grieves differently.

I invited Chris and Sandy to make their own special memory box about Grandma.

Chris brought in Grandma's favourite type of chocolate box which still had a strong 'chocolaty' smell; Grandma loved chocolates, so Chris said that felt right.

Developmentally the work needed to engage Chris on a concrete and physical level, where his memories of Grandma were 'easily perceived' (Bauchsbaum 1996: 117).

Chris made a 'garage' out of the box in which he placed a little red model car, which he had brought back from her flat. He said that he could use the car to travel in his mind to Chocolate Heaven, where he could see Grandma sitting in her armchair surrounded by boxes of chocolates!

Chris had located Grandma in a physical heaven that he could show us and talk about; his next step to holding onto a relationship with her.

Chris stuck photographs of Grandma and himself together, on the ceiling of the 'garage' and on the front, demonstrating his continued relationship with his grandma. 'Now Mummy will smile when she sees this', Chris told me proudly.

Through Chris's demonstration of how he could travel in his mind to see Grandma in 'Chocolate Heaven', the whole family was helped, by creating their healing stories about Grandma and their ongoing relationship with her. They shared experiences of mourning in terms of their own developmental perspectives, mother and sister adding stories about 'Grandma's sense of humour' which was 'passed on' to them. What death means to each is now witnessed in a supportive way by the other (Jones 2007: 102) and after six sessions they all reported feeling 'braver to talk' as a family. The teacher noticed that Chris appeared 'happier and calmer' at school.

Sensing our mother

Two sisters, who had lost both their parents in Africa, were now living in the UK with an aunt and her family. The aunt said Mary often appeared 'inconsolable' and she did not know how to make Mary feel better when she felt 'so bad' herself. The younger sister, Bea, was very quiet and withdrawn; life had been hard for this family for a very long time and coping mechanisms were already stretched. Their father had died of an Aids-related illness four years previously and then their mother died in a train crash. There had been changes of home and school before the journey to the UK. These extra stresses caused difficulties in the primary care giver's ability to respond to the children's attachment signals and feelings of inadequacy, leading to low self-esteem and despondency (Jewett 1997: 146).

Despite the school's efforts to include her, Mary, the eldest, sat alone in the playground and in class. The dramatherapy contract was 12 sessions with a recommendation that the aunt would see a counsellor from her GP surgery and join the girls in school-based sessions when she felt well enough. The family agreed that in order to support the girls through the therapy and in school, the therapist should liaise with the class teacher and they could each have a class 'buddy'.

Sensory work has long been incorporated into dramatherapy (Jennings 1995) and continues to be used in research into working through trauma (Lahad et al. 2010).

Mary and Bea sat with me on the 'story mat', gently touching and smelling the fruits that I had placed there. I asked them if some fruits smelt better than others. Mary chose the mango, talking about how she liked its sweet juice, so I suggested she bring it up to her face to inhale deeply.

Slowly, Mary shared an 'inner picture' of a memory of her and Bea eating a mango that their mother had given them. Mary smiled shyly at me across the mat and I suggested that this good feeling could be felt in her body and perhaps had a particular place and colour. 'It's here', she said, touching her chest, 'my heart . . . it's red and it's warm'.

If we help the client to focus on 'good sensations and emotional resources' says Lahad et al., we are equipping them for a journey into exposure of more distressing material (2010: 392).

The girls had said that they would like to try and recreate stories from 'back home', understanding that some would be difficult and others would hopefully bring more loving feelings back into their family life. The girls would explore their own story-making techniques through play with objects, writing, drawing and acting, each being a witness to the other. Following discussions, their aunt had brought in a selection of photographs from their life in Africa to use in this process.

On their fifth session, I asked them to select their most 'comforting' and their most 'uncomfortable' photograph. Some of the photographs contained images of people and places that the girls found distressing. The girls practised finding the 'safe' and 'loving' place inside them, which I asked them to 'sense' again, remembering the mango when they felt overwhelmed. Standing and shaking out their trembling arms and legs, running away from the photograph and back again, I invited them to write 'bubble' messages around the photograph.

I attempted to guide them to a place where they could find their relationship with their parents and acknowledge it with each other. The girls held strong Christian values, 'I hope God is looking after you', Bea wrote to her mother. Using sensory art materials, the girls made pictures of heaven. They wrote poems, which they performed to each other about their parents 'looking down on them'.

Outside the session, Mary included herself more in classroom activities and Bea spoke about how she could be included more in playground games. The girls decided that they wanted to share some of their stories from back home with their class. With Mary's class teacher's support, Mary also found the courage to read a story about her mother in an English lesson.

Mary was energised after she had shared something so personal about herself with her class. She had completed her task successfully without the therapist being present. Bea was encouraged by Mary's courage, saying 'Now I want people to know the real me.' As their dramatherapist, I accompanied them both into the class for this last shared ritual of transition, sharing their memory book of stories from back home with their class.

I believed that Mary and Bea had been struggling to hold onto a relationship with their parents and as Normand et al.'s research demonstrates, 'maintaining an interactive relationship' was paramount to the children's ability to cope (1996: 91).

Accepting that the deceased can be held in mind for children and that this relationship endures over time can extend the opportunity of coming back from loss and disconnectedness to relatedness.

A close bereavement will disrupt a child's inner and external world, but how that world is reconstructed will depend on the intervention offered to them. As dramatherapists our role is to act as facilitators and witnesses to the playing and telling of stories from the past, helping children and families to transform meaning for their future. This intervention enables children to reconnect with their lost relationship, so that they may both enjoy and achieve their full potential in school.

References

Abdelnoor, A. and Hollins, S. (2004) 'The effect of childhood bereavement on secondary school performance', *Educational Psychology in Practice*, 20 (1), 43–54.

Bauchsbaum, B. (1996) 'Remembering a parent who has died: A developmental perspective', in D. Klass, P. Silverman, and S. Nickman (eds.), *Continuing Bonds*. Philadelphia: Taylor and Francis.

Bowlby, J. (1980) *Attachment and Loss: Loss, Sadness and Depression*, Vol. 3. New York: Basic Books.

Cattanach, A. (1994) *Play Therapy: Where the Sky Meets the Underworld*. London: Jessica Kingsley.

Fauth, B., Thomson, M., and Penny, A. (2009) *Associations Between Childhood Bereavement and Children's Background, Experiences and Outcomes: Secondary analysis of the mental health of children and young people in Great Britain 2004 data*. London: NCB.

Fredman, G. (1997) *Death Talk: Conversations with Children and Families*. London: Karnac Books.

Gersie, A. (1996) *Storymaking in Bereavement*. London: Jessica Kingsley.

Jennings, S. (1995) 'Dramatherapy for survival', in S. Jennings (ed.), *Dramatherapy with Children and Adolescents*. London: Routledge.

Jewett, J. (1997) *Helping Children Cope with Separation and Loss*. London: Free Association Books.

Jones, P. (2007) *Drama as Therapy*, 2nd edn. London: Routledge.

Lahad, M., Farhi, M., Leykin, D., and Kapalansky, N. (2010) 'Preliminary study of a new integrative approach in treating post-traumatic stress disorder', *The Arts in Psychotherapy*, 37, 391–399.

Landy, R. (1996) *Essays in Drama Therapy*. London: Jessica Kingsley.

Normand, C., Silverman, P., and Nickman, S. (1996) 'Bereaved children's changing relationship with the deceased', in D. Klass, P. Silverman, and S. Nickman (eds.), *Continuing Bonds: New Understandings of Grief*. Philadelphia: Taylor & Francis.

Silverman, P. and Klass, D. (1996) Introduction: 'What's the problem?', in D. Klass, P. Silverman, and S. Nickman (eds.), *Continuing Bonds: New Understandings of Grief*. Philadelphia: Taylor & Francis.

Silverman, P. and Nickman, S. (1996) 'Children's construction of their dead parents', in D. Klass, P. Silverman, and S. Nickman (eds.), *Continuing Bonds*. Philadelphia: Taylor & Francis.

11 Education, the Playground Project and elements of psychodrama

Geoffrey Court, Jeffrey Higley and Olivia Lousada

The events described in this chapter took place in the early 1980s. It was a time when educational drama (Slade 1954) and drama therapy (Jennings 1973), as well as psychodrama, were taking their place amongst other developments in a movement towards the 'education of the whole person', and around which there was great excitement. But can a project that took place nearly 30 years ago be relevant now? Discussing this question at length, we the writers found ourselves looking beyond short-term utilitarianism, remembering that education is, among other things, an exploration into what it means to be human. Our project still seems to us both universal and timeless. We believe it represents an educational approach still being fought for in today's mainstream classroom – exemplified, indeed, by the publication of this book. In due course, a full account of the project may be published elsewhere. For now we offer a fragment based on an edited version of the record made at the time. We have kept as close as possible to the original text, adding some new reflections to facilitate the reader's understanding. All names have been changed.

Despite its title, The Playground Project happened in a classroom with a group of 23 children, aged 10–11 years old, and their teacher at a primary school on a deprived inner-city estate. Strong feelings, often reflected in the children's behaviour, were getting in the way of useful learning, and the teacher, Geoffrey Court, was looking for ways of addressing the problem. At that time Jeffrey Higley, a freelance performer, was working in the school as actor-in-residence, and he suggested that the psychodramatist Olivia Lousada might be able to help. The Playground Project was the result.

Like the project itself, the name originated through Olivia Lousada's experiences both as a professional and as a parent. She had been running a course for teachers who ran nurture groups, in which each session focused on a theme such as trust, power, or status. When the teachers tried out the material in the classroom, they were amazed to discover what was really going on in the peer group of the children: who liked whom, who stuck up for whom, how they felt about the bully in the class who felt he had no friends. This they learnt through the sociometry (the mapping of relationships). Olivia saw that the same insights might help her own six-year-old son, who was himself having a bad time in the playground. She knew that many children find the playground difficult and lonely, with a culture of its own. What if the energy of this peer group culture could be harnessed and used creatively? The implications of this question seemed enormous.

Sociometry of the peer group could become a tool for teachers

Our thinking was that sociometry of the peer group could become a tool for teachers, instead of the peer group being a challenge to their authority. The result could be 'children-centred' education alongside 'child-centred' education. What was needed was an approach that would allow the relationships between peers in the class to be examined, so that it became an educational tool. This was the rationale of the Playground Project.

The original project took the form of six fortnightly sessions of one and a half hours each, but the richness of the process meant that sessions soon had to be doubled in length, something more easily managed in the days before the National Curriculum. Broadly, the first four sessions each had a theme: 'Trust', 'Caring', 'Power', and 'Sabotage'. In the fifth session, the class was introduced to the Magic Shop, devised by Hannah Weiner (private communication with Marcia Karp), one of the first students to study psychodrama with J. L. Moreno. After this, the final session was designed as an opportunity to draw everything together before saying goodbye. We have chosen two of these sessions to describe in detail: the third session, 'Power', in which we ran into difficulties – from which much was learned – and the fifth session, 'the Magic Shop', which illustrates the access to creativity of this work.

Example one

Session 3: Power

The class teacher was absent. As a consequence of this the third session became a confrontation between different views of power, and therefore an enactment of the very theme we set out to explore. Our aim here is to give an honest account that raises questions about the relationship between containment and meaningful learning. It shows how adult assumptions, conscious and unconscious, can influence a classroom situation.

When Olivia and Jeffrey arrived they were told that Geoffrey, the class teacher, was absent, but they decided to continue nevertheless with their predetermined plan. This decision was to have huge consequences for children and adults alike, and it ultimately led to valuable insights. Most important, perhaps, was the understanding learnt that work of this kind, which involved breaking boundaries, depended absolutely on the safety and security provided by the presence of the trusted teacher.

Olivia and Jeffrey began by recalling the previous session ('Caring') and talking about 'taking care'. Several children offered examples:

> I shut my cat's tail in the door.
> My dog took care of me.

Wayne was very uneasy and there was a general climate of rising tension, shuffling and moving about. Jeffrey introduced the subject of the teacher's absence, and 90% of the children agreed they missed him and it was good to have someone big taking care. When we asked why, the children's answers all referred to the laying down of boundaries:

> "Geoffrey stops us fighting."
> "He looks after our money".
> "He counts us on the way to swimming".

Olivia and Jeffrey suggested that the children wanted them to be 'the teacher', which led to some discussion. At this point, either the two adults should have stopped the session, or one of them should have taken over the teacher's role. They could also have expanded on what this containment meant for the children, and how they could learn through experience to exercise it for themselves. None of these options was taken, however, since neither adult wanted the responsibility of the Teacher role. More positively, there was also a genuine wish to find new and different relational dynamics through which to foster teaching and learning.

So in the name of democratization, Olivia and Jeffrey decided to play the 'Yes Let's' game, in which one of the group says, 'Let's all . . .' and the rest respond 'Yes Let's' and perform the action until another person says, 'Let's all . . .'. The rule was that there should be no physical contact. Annie as usual relaxed and became excited by physical movement; her face really opened up in movement and situations where she could release her energy. Andrew seemed to need to bang into everyone despite the 'no contact' rule. The adults noticed his behaviour but did not confront it.

When break time came, most of the group wanted to stay in and continue the session. Three children disagreed: they wanted to go outside and practise football. Much discussion followed, with the children demanding that the adults should decide what was to happen, while the adults in turn wanted the class to make the decision. In an uneasy compromise, Jeffrey and Olivia ruled that those who went to break would later have to work outside so as not to disrupt proceedings. This was a strange decision in view of it being break time in the school. The adults saw it as a group decision; the children saw it as an adult decision. There was continual pressure, in the form of silly behaviour, for Olivia and Jeffrey to establish themselves as authority figures, but they continued to resist the role.

The next 'democratic' activity was an attempt to keep the children engaged with the theme of power through first-hand experience. They were asked to form a line according to size, with the biggest at one end and the smallest at the other. They were given no adult help and there was considerable argument. Adam was obviously at the head of the line and Sam at the end. Annie perceived herself several sizes larger than reality and became very angry when nobody else would agree with her. Finally she couldn't accept her position in the line and left the room. Knowing that she would be safe and supervised by other adults within the confines of the small classroom block, Jeffrey told her she was welcome to come back, but that it would be her decision. (She sneaked back in later.)

Adam and Sam were asked to face each other and each say something good about being the size of the other. Sam said that it would be good to be able to help people and protect them. Adam couldn't think of anything but then said, "It's too risky." He seemed to have no real awareness of what he had said, and the group was puzzled by his remark. This would have been fruitful to explore, especially as Wayne and the others who had left, ostensibly because they wanted to play football, had also remarked, "We're no good at this sort of thing, they don't want us anyway."

At this point, what with people from outside coming in to borrow rubbers, pencils and generally to make their presence felt, as well as the people inside stepping up the pressure, Jeffrey and Olivia had begun to feel that things were coming apart. Not knowing how else to manage the disorder, they gave everyone a classic 'sitting down and writing' task, still based on the 'power' theme: the children were to describe someone who made them feel smaller and someone who made them feel bigger. They then had to write one good thing about being big and one good thing about being small. This was generally thought about only in the physical sense, although one or two grasped the idea of non-physical size. Jeffrey picked up on this, talking about how big you feel in certain situations, and said that he felt fairly small at that moment. This intervention brought the question of authority to the fore, the dynamic shifted, and the class began to offer advice: 'Why don't you shout and tell us off?' Olivia and Jeffrey asked, 'Would that make us feel big?' 'Yes,' was the answer, 'it's got to, hasn't it?' At last, we were in a place of learning.

Teacher authority as oppression? Or as safe containment?

In this session the adults had made the mistake of allowing the 'rigid teacher' in their minds to take precedence. The central issue, Geoffrey's absence, was where the emotional energy of the group lay. This is where the focus of the session would have stayed, had Olivia and Jeffrey been able to respond more spontaneously. As it was, their responses came out of preconceptions (held by everyone, adults and children alike) based on an inhibiting idea of teacher authority as oppression, instead of teacher authority providing the safe containment that would enable the children to be creative. The adults had imposed activity so that something would seem to be being achieved. As a result, the group had gradually disintegrated.

Although Olivia and Jeffrey appeared to be the active leaders of the Playground Project, they realized after this session that the role of the teacher was paramount. It was the teacher, in the context of the school as a whole, who provided the containing environment that made possible a creative approach to problem-solving. The episode had illuminated a major tension that is part of a teacher's life, between the need for containment on the one hand and the need to remain emotionally available, as truthfully as possible, on the other. The ever-shifting relationship between safe containment and authentic emotional presence may be hard to manage, but any adult embarking on this kind of work, largely non-verbal as it is, has to grapple with the fact that disguising herself or himself makes it harder to perceive covert messages from others. Children, like adults, have a quite astounding capacity to know the truth of how we feel, and without emotional authenticity there can be no trust, therefore no creativity or learning.

Example two

Session 5: The Magic Shop

The fifth, penultimate session introduced The Magic Shop, an opportunity to dramatize and reformulate the energy behind emotional, social and academic learning. It focused attention on Charlie, seen by the group as its most isolated member. Charlie was at that time a third-year junior, small in stature and noticeably inhibited and wooden in his movements. In common with his younger brother and older sister, he usually wore a fixed smile, which others could find irritating. He was having difficulty in learning to read and write: he appeared too inhibited to work at all if other children were nearby, and his handwriting was too small to be legible. He rarely wrote more than two lines and before he could even produce this he had to screen himself behind an 'office' consisting of large folders standing on end.

Charlie sought special status by constantly mentioning, for example, the considerable age difference between his parents, or the fact that he had five Christian names. He knitted conspicuously and often sang loudly at inappropriate times. When the class sat down for a story, Charlie always had to be fetched, usually because he was obsessively tidying up. All this had helped to cut off Charlie from the rest of the children, some of whom treated him with amused tolerance, while others were openly scornful. It is hardly surprising that sometimes he seemed to be deeply unhappy. Virginia Axline reminds us that:

> Even though the group relationship seems to point up the problems and seems to hasten the development of insight, the responsibility to institute change remains with the child . . . Change in behaviour, if it is

to have any lasting value, must come from within the individual as a result of insight that he has achieved.

(Axline 1969: 106)

Thus it was that Charlie agreed to become the first visitor to the Magic Shop, which for our purposes took the following form. The class created an arena by sitting in a circle, and the shop, set by the children in Outer Space, came into being. The Magic Shop sells qualities and feelings in different-sized bottles and packs. These imaginary goods can exist as soaps, shampoos, drinks or in any other form, and may be taken or applied as appropriate. In order to pay for their requirements, shoppers must contribute a feeling – something they wish to have less of or be rid of – to the mixture in the shopkeeper's cauldron, so that it can be recycled for someone who could use some of it. All the other children in the class become the packages, bottles or jars and choose the size and quality that they wish to be. They also choose the form of the remedy (tablet, ointment, drink and so on) that they feel is suitable to the shopper's needs.

Jeffrey supported Charlie throughout the exercise, acting as his 'double' in order to magnify his actions and thought. 'The function of the double is to help give expression to the deepest emotions of the protagonist. The double supports the protagonist so gradually he can take more risks and enter into the interaction more completely. The double can also give effective suggestions and interpretations to the protagonist which can be accepted or rejected' (Blatner 1973: 24).

Geoffrey consulted Charlie about how he was going to arrive at the shop. Charlie decided he was going to fly in a mouse rocket. After his arrival Olivia, as shopkeeper, asked what she could do for him. What was his problem? After some hesitation he said that he had a very stiff leg. In fact his legs and hips were very stiff and he walked about like a robot. Olivia questioned him; did this stiffness stop him doing things? Yes, football and joining in. Olivia positioned herself very close to him and asked if the stiffness was anywhere else. It was also on his chest. How was he to get rid of this stiffness? Some of the group suggested he fight it out. In the end he decided to shake it out. At first he worked gingerly, but with Olivia's encouragement he became deeply involved and worked intensely, gripping the attention of everyone in the class. Jeff worked alongside Charlie, shaking and moving with him until he felt released from his stiffness.

Charlie next decided he needed a membership potion to drink and used two people, one as a glass and one as a bottle, which was very amusing for everyone. The opportunity to receive help, and to give it, made him quite elated and he offered people rides in his spaceship. We said it was extendable and could take a great many people, and there was a grand procession around the room.

A 'sharing' session followed, with many children falling over themselves to have the next turn. Some were angry at being among the last to board

Charlie's spaceship: this in itself could have become the subject of further exploration.

Over subsequent months the Magic Shop was to become a regular gathering place and the main point of reference in the shared culture of the group. The controlled framework into which these symbols emerge has much in common with ritual. There are certain boundaries to be observed which create the safety necessary for freedom of expression, and an arena into which each individual could come for support. The shop became a safe, bounded space that made the children's imaginative empathy and generosity of spirit more immediately available. The group could be a resource to itself. By extension, it also became a place where conflict could be resolved and, crucially, where the continuing 'story' of classroom life could be told.

In the Magic Shop, myth, symbol and ritual fused with spontaneous performance to create an authentic theatre of the heart. All children literally inhabit the world of myth and fairytale, surrounded without by adult giants and powerful seemingly magic or demonic forces within. The power of these forces is encapsulated by Bettelheim in his groundbreaking study on the conscious and unconscious meaning of fairy stories in *The Uses of Enchantment* (1976). Outwardly children exist, often bewildered, in a landscape and a society they did not create and cannot control and yet will inevitably inherit. Often, because of the pressure of time, money, family and circumstances, they become victims of threatening, monstrous figures, images of past failures, of fragments of locked-away, half-admitted elements of the self. Such tormentors inevitably slow or paralyse learning or achievement. These problems find vivid and concrete expression in the myth of the heroic quest, the symbol of the journey to the centre of the labyrinth.

The symbols in a psycho-dramatic story can be both intensely personal and universal at the same time. Symbols and reality can be very close; perhaps children distinguish between the two even less than adults do. As more visitors came in turn to the Magic Shop, it was frequently surprising how an apparently slight image or object could grow in stature and significance. This was true for the group as well as for the individual: in fact, at times it seemed that the group was more in touch than the main protagonist – the main actor – with the meaning of a symbol. Perhaps the difference was that while the image might not be new to the protagonist, the group was always taken by surprise. Their attention was caught. This was reflected in the enthusiasm of the group for the Magic Shop. The effect was greatest when physical involvement and action were level with dialogue: when we dropped into pure discussion, the level of engagement dropped correspondingly.

The value of spontaneity

It was and remains quite apparent that where people feel they can be spontaneous in their relationships, this in turn fosters creativity in their other learning. Creativity, 'the highest form of intelligence' (J. L. Moreno 1977: XII), is described by Zerka Moreno as a 'sleeping beauty' (2006: 208) awoken by spontaneity. Spontaneity is the capacity to find a new response to an old situation, or an appropriate response to a present situation and therefore the future. In this project, spontaneity facilitated the creativity and learning of the whole group. Blatner 'points out that our civilisation has relegated . . . to childhood spontaneity, creativity and play . . . Children understand symbolism very well . . . (They also) understand that most adults have lost the ability to play and . . . to understand symbolism' (Bannister 1991: 80). This chapter in this book is a plea for the beauty of the lived and learned experience as part of education.

Kipper encapsulated the psycho-dramatic position, 'Human beings are born actors . . . (They) master the world that surrounds them' (1986: 3). Through the mastery of many roles and spontaneity, the self also emerges. Spontaneity is about being in the 'here and now' (Williams 1989: 12). It delights us to see this in children who know no other way to be. So it follows that recognition of the prime importance of the body and of 'experiencing reality as a means to change (and learning) rather than just talking through' (Marineau 1989: 49) needs to be valued in education. Moreno held 'well-being and spontaneity go hand in hand' (cited in Lousada 2009: 41). Spontaneity and creativity in turn naturally lead to reflection that facilitates the internalization of the lived and learned experience in all aspects of social, emotional, creative and academic education.

In the classroom we as teachers mostly concern ourselves, rightly, with the learning of the individual child; however, this work was concerned just as much with the learning of the group. A class can be stuck with a reputation, just as an individual can, and like an individual it can learn to change. Of course, the Magic Shop was not really magic, and life in that classroom, where so many of the children were leading deeply troubled lives, continued sometimes to be difficult. There can be no doubt though that this was significant for all concerned, and when we, the writers, came together again, we were all astonished and delighted to discover how fresh the work still felt, and how vividly we remembered it. It belongs not in our past, but in our present.

Appendix

Psychodrama, sociometry, the social atom, sociograms and Tele

Amongst his many inventions J.L. Moreno (1890–1974) saw psychodrama as the supreme contribution. In his philosophy he saw man as warming up to action and this manifested itself spontaneously in the quest for new solutions and creativity in every aspect of life, as well as in the here and now. He was interested in changing communities and saw man's greatest gift as spontaneity and creativity.

Psychodrama and dramatherapy

Psychodrama means the drama of the psyche. This refers to the relationship world created from lived experiences and how we internalize these experiences to keep ourselves alive, that in turn informs our choices. For example, when we feel pleased with something we have done and then we criticize it brutally, there is an internal struggle of relationships that may be invented roles or internalized relationships from those experienced in life. Psychodrama is *not* role-play. Role-play is a made-up situation. Psychodrama is a person's real internal story represented by objects or people as the individual experiences them, so the individual can explore their dilemma in a concrete way. This means that their experience is represented outside them so they can look at it, walk around it, and experience it from different points of view, to help them find out what is missing and unexpressed, and to gain a new response. Dramatherapy is based in the meaning-making of metaphor through the arts, whilst psychodrama is based in the metaphor of the internal world and the emergent meaning of the drama of the psyche. The interchange between these two methods is beautifully close and mirrors different levels of meaning-making that facilitate spontaneity, creativity and change. The essence of this is seen in the Magic Shop, in which the external structure is a creative imagined space – that is, dramatherapy in style – whilst the process is created through the representation of the boy's struggle with what he personally has to give up in order to find a new role. This is psychodramatic. Many dramatherapists use aspects of psychodrama, as psychodramatists use aspects of dramatherapy.

The tools of psychodrama

Whilst only some aspects of psychodrama are seen in the work described here, the underlying philosophy was present in the approach through spontaneity and creativity. The aim of psychodrama is to restore spontaneity. 'Spontaneity' here does not mean impulsiveness but 'a new response to old situations, or an adequate response to a present or future situation'. In this context, tools of psychodrama employed were:

'The director'.
'The warming up' or preparation of the group towards the work.
'The double', the role of support.
'The protagonist', the one who is in need of help.
'The auxiliary egos', the role of the others.
'The sharing' of the group as to how they identify with the protagonist. Sharing helps the protagonist rejoin the group by finding that they are not alone in what they feel. It helps the group identify important learning for themselves.

This list is not prescriptive. Other 'tools' could have been used:

'Role reversal' or stepping into the role of the other.
'Mirroring', the standing back by the protagonist to look at him/herself in the whole story.

To help spontaneity in the group, there is a preparation or warming up to the task and being present in the moment through activity or discussion. This may be done through sociometry.

Sociometry, the social atom, sociometric choice and Tele

Sociometry is a method of measuring and evaluating group dynamics through action, written statements or questionnaires. This can be conducted in a mathematical large community exercise, but here it simply refers to the expression of choice by each person to another person in the group. This can be done by placing a hand on the shoulder of choice or standing beside the person of their choice.

Sociometric theory involves three basic concepts: the social atom, sociometric choice, and Tele. The social atom is the network of an individual's relationships, be they social, emotional or cultural that emerge through Tele. These networks are always changing and adjusting in life.

Tele is seen in the emotional tension of attraction, repulsion and indifference emerging in a group. These responses can be recorded as a sociogram or map of relationships of the individual, or as a sociometric map that records the choices of a group rather than an individual. Tele is the insight into and ability to assume the feelings of the other. Tele is what makes for a more harmonious, secure and lively group. It has also been found that if an individual finds more fulfilment in less intimate groups (e.g. work or school groups), this may produce changes in his more intimate group (family). The relationships of Tele in the playground are therefore paramount in the experience of social, emotional, creative and educational dimensions for each child in the school, and the groups she or he inhabits.

Acknowledgement

The authors wish to acknowledge the kindness of Marcia Karp.

References

Axline, V.M. (1969) *Play Therapy*. New York: Ballantine Books/Random House.
Bannister, A. (1991) 'Learning to live again', in P. Holmes and M. Karp (eds.), *Inspiration and Technique*. London: Routledge.
Bettelheim, B. (1976) *The Uses of Enchantment*. New York: Random House.
Blatner, H.A. (1973) *Acting-In*. New York: Springer.

Jennings, S. (1973) *Remedial Drama*. London: Pitman.
Kipper, D.A. (1986) *Psychotherapy Through Clinical Role Playing*. New York: Brunner/Mazel.
Lousada, O. (2009) *Hidden Twins*. London: Karnac.
Marineau, R.F. (1989) *Jacob Levy Moreno*. London: Routledge.
Moreno, J.L. (1977) *Psychodrama, First Volume*. New York: Beacon House.
Moreno, Z. (2006) *The Quintessential Zerka*. T. Horvatin and E. Schreiber (eds.). New York: Routledge.
Slade, P. (1954) *Child Drama*. London: University of London Press.
Williams, A. (1989) *The Passionate Technique*. London: Routledge.

12 Beginning, middle, end, beginning: dramatherapy with children who have life-limiting conditions and with their siblings

Alyson Coleman and Alison Kelly

> A well rounded life should have a beginning, middle and end.
>
> (Murray Parkes 1970: vi)

This chapter will focus on a dramatherapy intervention with two children – a boy with a life-limiting condition and his sister. Jason and Sophie are a constructed case (Yalom 1980), but the vignettes contain patterns and themes that have emerged from actual sessions. There will be reference to dramatherapy and child bereavement theories, which underpin the practice. The work takes place within an NHS Children's Bereavement Service that was specifically established to support children who have life-limiting conditions and their siblings.

> The term life-limiting refers to a medical condition for which there is no reasonable hope of cure.
>
> (Association for Children with Life-threatening or Terminal Conditions and Their Families, ACT 2003)

The dramatherapy forms part of a holistic approach to children's palliative care within a community health service. The therapy fits with the ethos of palliative care defined by ACT as it 'embraces physical, emotional, social and spiritual elements and focuses on enhancement of quality of life for the child/young person' (ACT 2003). In addition to substantial dramatherapy experience with children in specialist and mainstream education, the therapists have further training in childhood bereavement through gaining a postgraduate certificate from St Christopher's Hospice Education Centre and Help the Hospices, London. Dramatherapy is supported within a framework of individual, joint, team supervision and external consultation.

The method of combining co-facilitation with siblings and individual work has developed organically within the service. Sessions with a therapist who has a relationship with the sibling before their death has enhanced all the post-bereavement sibling work the service has offered.

Examples of referrals within one family

Jason Smith

Age: Eleven years
Referrer: Head of Year, Special Educational Needs School

Reason for referral

Jason seems very unhappy at school. He gets frustrated and angry with staff and other children. He has deteriorated physically, and is finding writing, computers, anything to do with his hands, very difficult. His mobility in general has become significantly impaired. He seems isolated and withdrawn. The staff are concerned that he is keeping his fears and questions about dying to himself.

Background information

Jason was diagnosed with a life-limiting, degenerative condition at a young age. The dramatherapy took place at the Special Educational Needs School that he attends, after he transferred from mainstream school because of his medical needs. He lives at home with regular short breaks at the children's hospice.

Sophie Smith

Age: Nine years
Referrer: Head of Year, Special Educational Needs School

Reason for referral

'Mrs Smith mentioned to the nurses that she is worried about Sophie, who is complaining of tummy aches in the mornings and not wanting to go to school. She has become very "clingy" to her mum.'

Background information

Sophie has grown up knowing that Jason has special medical needs. Nurses and hospitals have always been a part of family life. She has seen his health deteriorate and notices his loss of mobility and changing body.

Family information

The Smith family are Church of England, white British, with no underlying physical or mental health difficulties. Grandparents and an aunt live nearby and there are no major difficulties in the respective families of origin. The family home has been adapted for Jason's needs. They have a good collaborative working relationship with health, education and social services. Mr Smith is in full-time work, Mrs Smith works part-time.

Rhythms of sessions within the service vary according to the specific circumstances of the children. Initially there may be weekly sessions followed by less frequent appointments and then a return to a more intense intervention at times of crisis or change. A child may be affected by their condition for a long period of time, often years, so the service has developed sustainable ways of 'holding' the therapeutic process with the child or young person. The child is then able to draw upon this work when needed, knowing that there will be more sessions on specific dates in the future.

Following an initial assessment with the Smith family and information gathering from the health and education professionals involved, dramatherapy sessions commenced within two weeks. A working alliance was established (Hawkins and Shohet 2000). The dramatherapists were involved with the family for a two-year period in total, before and after Jason's death.

Jason had a combination of weekly and fortnightly sessions at school, at the hospice and at home, including three joint sessions with Sophie several months before he died.

The children worked with the Japanese story of *The Chestnut Tree* in shared and individual sessions (Singh and Cann 2003).

The story is about a young girl whose father dies at sea; to support her ageing mother, the girl has to find work in a town far away. During the daily journey she befriends a beautiful chestnut tree, who offers her comfort and strength over many years. She tells herself it was a bad dream when the tree informs her that it is to be cut down and made into a boat for the prince and it is time for them to part. The tree instructs her to come and find the boat, which will not move until she is reunited with it. One day during a big storm she runs for shelter, only to discover that her beloved tree is indeed gone and it had spoken the truth. She weeps and collects chestnut leaves to remind her of her friendship with the tree. Life was never the same again. One day in the town she sees the prince attempting in vain to launch his fine new boat in front of all of the town's people. As the tree had predicted, the boat would not be moved until the young girl came and whispered words of greeting and touched the chestnut wood. The crowd falls silent witnessing this moment.

Individual dramatherapy with Jason

Jason was particularly drawn to the part of the story when the girl discovers the tree has gone. He objected strongly to the fact that the story did not give the detail of what happened to the tree. Where had it gone? He accused the therapist of 'forgetting' that part, getting it 'wrong' and 'not telling that bit on purpose'.

Over many sessions Jason brought several contrasting versions of what may have happened to the tree, which were enacted with the therapist. Worden (1996) suggests that children will fantasize about illness and death if they are not given age-appropriate information. Enactment enabled Jason to explore his thoughts and fears, which previously he had felt unable to share verbally.

Vignette

Jason becomes the prince. The prince is very powerful and arrogant. He treats his servants very badly, calling them useless and stupid. The dramatherapist is directed to become one of the servants, who is humiliated by the prince. Jason directs the therapist in this role to become more and more incapable – the servant drops the food and drink he is serving, he does not get the jokes the prince tells him, he is too slow to catch the prince's very expensive horse that runs off and is lost.

This session seemed to be about actual loss of bodily function and independence in the present. This aspect of the condition was incredibly difficult for Jason to deal with. It affected each and every relationship. His family, friends and school staff responded in different ways – from obvious distress to denial. Observing him daily losing the ability to grip objects, speak and move was so difficult for him and others that he became very isolated.

The child's emotional and spiritual maturity may contrast sharply with their physical limitations and lack of independence. As a toddler, Jason ran, moved and played. He remembers this somatically, cognitively and emotionally.

The part of the story Jason chose to create and enact enabled him to explore being the master and the servant. The prince may have represented his illness, which is often 'in charge', and the servant represented the functioning part of him that endeavours to carry on and get things done. The servant is capable but restricted by the prince's demands and limitations.

Dramatherapy has the potential to move and change quickly. Through the spontaneity of drama, the therapist can attempt to keep up and accompany the child with the rapid changes of feelings and perspectives that emerge from their process.

> A child can soar like a bird to experience a freedom she'll never know or a child can become death itself in order to face her darkest fears.
>
> (Bouzoukis 2001: 229)

Dramatherapy enabled Jason to embody a range of conflicting archetypes (Jung 1964). Within Jason's solo journey, he was able to create a landscape where friends and foes could battle and engage in dialogue. This appeared to lessen his isolation at a meaningful level as his impossible-to-voice fears and questions were brought into the creative work. On several occasions this included directly talking about his death, his life and his legacy.

Individual dramatherapy with Sophie

Sophie was in year 5 at the local primary school. Jason also attended this school until he transferred to a special educational needs school that could accommodate his physical and medical condition. Both dramatherapists met with Sophie's teacher and Special Educational Needs Co-ordinator (SENCO). Rowling (2003) acknowledges the importance of school as a community that provides security and continuity. At times of emotional change it can offer comfort and healing.

The dramatherapy work with Sophie offered her support with the actual daily experience of Jason's deteriorating health and also looked towards the future. The therapeutic relationship was maintained through different phases of Sophie's experience. Dramatherapy sessions can provide an opportunity to explore the theme of maximizing life in the face of death. In Sophie's individual pre-bereavement dramatherapy sessions she had been able to express her feelings of anger, embarrassment and confusion about her brother's condition, and worries and questions about his increasing disability. In their joint sessions, Sophie had been able to share some of her questions and fears with Jason. Over time, in her post-bereavement sessions, she was able to explore the theme of developing a new relationship with Jason (Klass et al. 1996).

After Jason's death the school requested staff training from the bereavement service. Silverman (2003: 19) suggests that effective support strategies can increase resilience in the grieving school community. There was anxiety amongst staff about what to say to Sophie and how to respond to questions from her peers. The therapists delivered the training before Sophie's return to school. Teachers and school staff can be a valuable resource for children when death affects a school community (Dyregrov 1991).

The session offered practical ways to support the children and was an opportunity for the entire staff, teaching and non-teaching members, many of whom had also known Jason since his first day at primary school, to share their memories and grief. The therapists spoke to the Head Teacher about risk assessment in terms of other children and staff for whom Jason's death might have a significant impact. Both Capewell (1994) and Yule (1993) emphasize how previous deaths are relevant to their responses to current losses.

During the first session after Jason's death, this was acknowledged by the dramatherapist. They also discussed the death at the hospice and when the funeral would be. For many children it can be a relief to know what information the adults have about their situation. Clarity around communication forms an essential part of the working alliance. Gersie (1987) supports the idea that children need to know how the therapist will liaise with other significant people in their life.

Vignette

'Jason knew he was going to die'.

Sophie told the therapist that her parents had explained to her that sometimes Jason had been very ill and got better, but this time the doctors and nurses could not make him better.

She said that sometimes when she woke up in the mornings before he died she used to tell herself that she had imagined it or made it up.

The therapist said that it reminded her of the story of *The Chestnut Tree* that they had worked with in several joint sessions with Jason towards the end of his life. There is the part where the tree tells the young girl that it is to be cut down and warns her that they will be parted. The girl tells the tree, 'I had a bad dream, I dreamed that the prince had given orders to cut you down.'

Sophie said that she didn't remember that part and asked the therapist to tell her the story again. She wrapped some fabrics around herself and put a large piece of lycra over her head and was very still as she listened to the story. Then together they retold the story using the parts that Sophie remembered. The therapist invited her to enact some of the story. She chose the part where the prince gives his orders for the tree to be cut down, but said, 'I don't want to hear the words'.

The therapist was directed to be the prince and Sophie chose to be a guard. They enacted that moment from the story. The therapist asked if Sophie wanted to swap roles; she did not want to. She requested to repeat that part three times; she gave the therapist instructions on how much emotion the prince was to show. The first two attempts were 'not angry enough!' She was able to use her body for the therapist to mirror the movements of the prince and the look on his face (Jones 1996).

Sophie then wanted to enact the same part, but this time she asked to be the girl sleeping and the therapist to be the prince, again giving the order to cut the tree down using words and sounds. They repeated this several times and then she got up from her 'sleeping' position and started to bang the drum and shake the rain stick, getting louder and louder until the prince's voice could not be heard. She put all the drums in the middle of the room and told the therapist 'you aren't the prince anymore, you're the forest, we are the forest and we hate the prince! We have to make the storm so loud that no one can hear the prince'.

There followed a lengthy period of banging and crashing of drums, cymbals and rain sticks, where she was able to articulate strong emotions with the use of sound, percussion and embodiment. Using sound can enable children to access emotions and embody them where words are inadequate or hard to find (Watts 1996).

'The tree was trying to warn her. That's the end for today', said Sophie, as she was putting on her shoes to go back to class.

During this session Sophie had found a way to embody her anger and to symbolically pose philosophical questions: Why does this have to happen? Why did Jason die? The story provided a container for her overwhelming range of emotions and supported her to integrate the healthy process of oscillating (Stroebe and Schut 1996) between restoration and loss. As Stokes (1997) observes, this may happen more rapidly for children than adults.

The Dual Process Model (Stroebe and Schut 1996) introduces the concept of oscillation between those coping behaviours that focus on the loss and those that focus on the future, with both being important for adaptation and finding new meaning in the loss. It is a framework that is an important part of theoretical underpinning within the dramatherapy bereavement work. It is also used as part of an assessment for a healthy, self-regulating bereavement process. It is derived from empirical research that concluded that avoiding grief may be both helpful and detrimental. To manage daily life Sophie needed to take time off from the emotions of grief, which may otherwise be too overwhelming (Worden 1991).

Sophie returned to the weekly pattern of dramatherapy sessions for a term at school. At the end of this period a dramatherapy report was written for school. Several follow-up visits were then booked in advance with Sophie and her family over the next few months. Regular telephone conversations took place with her teacher to offer informal support and guidance.

Conclusion

This chapter has looked at how dramatherapy can support children with life-limiting conditions and their siblings. With reference to vignettes from pre- and post-bereavement work, it has offered examples of how dramatherapy can work with feelings that may be difficult to share through words.

The original reasons for referral were explored through the use of story. Jason was able to work through feelings around his changing stages of physical ability and regain some control during a period of his life when he felt disempowered. Sophie gained space for herself and was able to build resilience at a time when her feelings were overwhelming and frightening. The therapists offered ongoing support and training to both schools involved with the children.

In this constructed case, the Dual Process Model (Stroebe and Schut 1996) combined with dramatherapy to take into account the individuality and diversity of grief. It encompasses the social, behavioural and spiritual dimensions of loss as well as the psychological and physical.

In his paper 'Mourning and Melancholia', Freud (1917) suggested that 'incomplete mourning as a child would make one vulnerable to adult depression'. The Child Bereavement Study (Worden 1996) researched the long-term consequences (after two years) of parental death for children. There is further research documented by Worden (1996) to suggest that some children who experience bereavement continue to develop mental health difficulties in adulthood. Although there are many questions still to be answered about these links, it remains clear that children do experience distress due to loss and that this may have a profound impact on their emotional and physical development into adulthood. Within the bereavement service, dramatherapy intervention has supported children on the edge of school exclusion, acting out difficult behaviours, extreme risk taking and eating difficulties. Dramatherapy has accompanied them through the intensity and unpredictable nature of illness and grief.

The focus of the therapists on life rather than on death enables the work to breathe and thrive. It does not ignore the truth, rather it aims to integrate all aspects of life and death in one human life cycle, which has a beginning, middle, end and beginning.

References

Association for Children with Life-threatening or Terminal Conditions and Their Families (2003) *A Guide to the Development of Children's Palliative Care Services*. The Association for Children with Life-threatening or Terminal Conditions and Their Families & Royal College of Paediatrics and Child Health. Available at: www.act.org.uk (Accessed 10 December 2010).

Bouzoukis, C.E. (2001) *They Couldn't Walk So They Learned To Fly*. London: Jessica Kingsley.

Capewell, E. (2004) *Working with Disaster. Transforming Experience into Useful Practice*. Doctoral thesis. University of Bath.

Dyregrov, A. (1991) *Grief in Children. A Handbook for Adults*. London: Jessica Kingsley.

Freud, S. (1917) 'Mourning and Melancholia'. *The Standard Edition of the Complete Psychological Works of Sigmund Freud* (Vol. XIV). London: Vintage, The Hogarth Press and the Institute of Psycho-Analysis.

Gersie, A. (1987) *Dramatherapy Theory and Practice for Teachers and Clinicians*. London: Routledge.

Hawkins, P. and Shohet, R. (2000) *Supervision in the Helping Professions*. Maidenhead: Open University Press.

Jones, P. (1996) *Drama as Therapy, Theatre as Living*. London: Routledge.

Jung, C.G. (1964) *Man and His Symbols*. London: Doubleday.

Klass, D., Silverman, P.R., and Nickman, S.L. (eds.) (1996) *Continuing Bonds*. London: Routledge.

Murray Parkes, C. (1970) 'Foreword', in E. Kubler-Ross, On Death and Dying. London: Tavistock.

Rowling, L. (2003) *Grief in School Communities*. Buckingham: Open University Press.

Silverman, P.R. (2003) *Never Too Young To Know: Death in Children's Lives*. New York: Oxford University Press.

Singh, R. and Cann, H. (2003) *A Forest of Stories*. Cambridge, MA: Barefoot Books.

St Christopher's Hospice Education Centre, Help the Hospices, London. Available at www.stchristophers.org.uk (Accessed 5 December 2010).

Stokes, J.A. (1997) *Then, Now and Always. Supporting Children as they Journey Through Grief: A Guide for Practitioners*. London: Calouste Gulbenkian Foundation.

Stroebe, M.S. and Schut, H. (1996) *A Model for Coping with Grief and its Practical Applications for the Bereavement Counsellor*. Paper presented at the third St George's 'Dying, Death and Bereavement' conference. St George's Hospital Medical School, London. 6 March 1996.

Watts, P. (1996) *Discovering the Self Through Drama and Movement*. London: Jessica Kingsley.

Worden, J.W. (1991) *Grief Counseling and Grief Therapy*. New York: Springer.

Worden, J.W. (1996) *Children and Grief*. New York: Guildford Press.

Yalom, I.D. (1980) *Existential Psychotherapy*. New York: Basic Books.

Yule, W. (1993) *Wise Before the Event*. London: Calouste Gulbenkian Foundation.

Part III

Collaborative partnerships in schools and beyond

13 Learning disabilities and finding, protecting and keeping the therapeutic space

Josephine Roger

This chapter is taken from a paper presented at the British Association of Dramatherapists Conference 'Dramatherapy in Education Now' on 1 July 2000.

My contribution to the discussion about dramatherapy in education is not so much about how we introduce dramatherapy into education, but much more about what happens when we do. I will concentrate on three main issues within this chapter.

The first issue is about the compatibility of the aims of the institution as a whole and that of the dramatherapy being practised. Compatibility needs to be the subject of continuous debate. In raising this issue I will be urging dramatherapists to remain as alert to unconscious communications as they are to spoken or written agreements because institutions, no less than individuals, develop defences against painful emotions. The nature of the work can give rise to anxieties, which need to be pushed away and denied (Obholzer and Roberts 1994: 137).

Secondly, there is the issue of the objectives of dramatherapy with a particular client group. I will argue that there are many ways to offer dramatherapy within an educational setting and there can be many different objectives set. What is important is that the objectives are clear and that they are shared with the teaching staff and teaching teams. The negotiation about the objectives will hopefully result in a genuine permission for the young people to come to use the therapy. This permission is needed so that young people can feel safe and make use of the therapy space. Even where there is common agreement about this and a partnership is formed between the therapist and teacher, it is important to remember that the work can be painful.

The third and most important issue I want to raise is why I feel that dramatherapy is useful within an educational setting. I cannot overstate my own belief that the provision of a therapeutic space for young people within their educational setting is of enormous value. The value of the therapeutic space is not confined to the actual therapy sessions themselves. Providing therapy within education provides an opportunity for staff to think about young people in a different and hopefully useful way. Sharing the work of the therapy will entail opening up discussion about issues such as personal and emotional development, group dynamics and the unconscious influences at work within the individual, the group and the institution. Having the opportunity to think together can help to make sense of the young people's behaviour. For example, thinking about the ambivalent feelings experienced by adolescents as they strive for independence and talking together about the dismissive and aggressive feelings this stirs up can help us to remember the sadness, remorse and fear of loss and rejection that is part and parcel of adolescence (Waddell 2002: 148).

Taking time to think about how dilemmas common to the age group affect the very different personal situations of young people helps to make sense of the way young people are managing the demands within the classroom.

It is helpful to make time to think about such issues. This does not mean that it is easy. In my experience, bringing things to mind is often a very painful process. There will be resistance to this. In the words of Valerie Sinason, 'Ignorance is not bliss and neither is knowledge' (Sinason 1992: 87).

However, the firm belief of those of us who strive for a place for dramatherapy within education is that if difficult and unbearable feelings can be brought to mind and named, then the consequence is a significant development in terms of a person's ability to think and to learn (Harris Williams 1987: 100–101).

I will illustrate these three points using my work as a dramatherapist in a college of further education. The work was with young people who were attending a range of special needs courses.

The institution and the therapy – finding a space

The question 'Is there space for dramatherapy within this institution?' was literally acted out in finding a physical space for the therapy within the college. We started off in the old, disused gym next door to the newly equipped drama studio. There was a notion then that we needed a large space and that we were allied to drama. I would say that the value of what we offered was under question. Perhaps the place of this client group, in terms of the priorities of a further education setting, was uncertain in the mind of the institution as a whole. A disused area next to a brand new studio provides a sharp contrast, which cannot help but raise a question.

A year later we were moved to the communication block. We were given the drama room, which had been vacated as a result of the new drama studio being built. This was a large space, with raised dais, but unfortunately it was sited directly above a language laboratory where silence was important. Though an ideal space in itself, in terms of the institution as a whole our placement here caused conflict. It raised the issue of what counts as learning.

Another year on and we were moved to the conference room, the special room of the college. It was used to host ad hoc conferences and special meetings. The value ascribed to the therapy and to the client group itself within this educational institution seemed to be more certain. The point I should have understood all along is the inextricable connection between our obvious increase in value within the institution and the support and backing of the senior management team. It was only much later that I learned how significant the principal's role was in providing and maintaining a space for dramatherapy within the institution. At the time, the allocation of such a special room provided me with a fairly high-profile presence. It provided me, as a dramatherapist, with what felt like a constant battle with staff, i.e. those in charge of scheduling rooms, heads of faculty and the vice-principals, in order to maintain the therapy time and space within this special room. What it also provided, of course, was a constant dialogue between the institution and myself at all sorts of level. As a result of this dialogue we achieved a clearer understanding of what dramatherapy was and what sort of space it needed.

We were next given a large room between the college's playgroup/crèche and the individual counselling room situated within the advice and guidance block. This felt like the clearest confirmation that the college had found a space for dramatherapy and that we had established, through dialogue, a clearer understanding of what dramatherapy was.

It was after a merger proposal, a change of Principal and a very definite change of ethos that the place of dramatherapy within the institution changed. We were finally placed, before our eventual demise, in the converted toilet block. To say now that I should have seen the writing on the wall is cruel but apt.

In the end, the work finished. No one ever said there is no space for dramatherapy within this institution. Instead there was a literal acting out of the fact that no space could be found and no room could be made for it. It was not enough that the course team fought for the therapy. The management team could not find a place for it within the now newly merged college.

The aims of the institution and of the therapy were no longer compatible. One of my errors, in this very large institution, was in focusing mainly on the relationship with the course tutor, at the expense of the management team. The management structure within the college changed several times and when posts were being merged and new people were being appointed only my meetings with the tutor remained regular. In times of transition and change the dialogue needs to be more active. The irony is that at such times of change and upheaval, energy is so easily focused upon survival, upon maintaining and protecting the space you have.

When dramatherapy is introduced into education a dialogue begins, but that dialogue needs to remain continuous and, at times of change and transition, become more vigorous.

The sort of therapy you offer and the forging of a partnership: it is still painful

I will use a piece of work I did with one particular group to illustrate this next point. The group consisted of eight young people who had learning disabilities and the work took place over a two-year period.

The young people were aged between 17 and 21. Some were visibly or obviously disabled in learning and some were more physically disabled. Some were able to talk, and some to read and write to a limited extent. Others were able to use one or two words but mainly communicated non-verbally. I saw the group once a week for a 90-minute session.

There are many ways of practising dramatherapy within educational settings. My way was shaped by the fact that I was offering relatively long-term work and that my clients had very particular needs. I saw the task as providing a space where the young people could explore and express what it meant to be adolescents with a learning disability. To tackle this task, which at times was very painful, meant that it was vital to be in dialogue with the tutor. My sense was that before the young people were really able to make use of the therapy, they had to test the strength and quality of the relationship between the therapist and the tutor. In the early days of the group, they would take issues from the session to be sorted by the tutor. They would do something on the way to or from the session, or they would say that they did not want to come to the session or they would refuse to leave. These were significant tests to the boundaries between therapy and teaching, but also were a direct challenge to the nature of the relationship between the two.

Being able to talk together about the meaning of this behaviour as tutor and therapist, and being clear about our respective roles in relation to the young people, was vital to the therapeutic work. My belief is that the young people will test what sort of parental couple the tutor and therapist are. They will test how safe a therapy space is.

The task of seeing things for what they are, that is, any form of disillusionment, is a difficult task for any of us. We have to feel safe to be able to tackle it. Bion (1970) talks about the struggle between the desire to know and understand the truth of one's own experience, on the one hand, and having a dread of knowing and understanding on the other. But what does this begin to mean if you are born different and possibly damaged? Sinason writes eloquently about the nature of learning disability. In terms of growing up she uses the game of King of the Castle to express one of the dilemmas:

> You are either the king of the castle or the stupid rascal. The two-year-old is murderously desperate to be king because otherwise he will have to face the fact that he is only tiny. The omnipotent adult or child with a handicap will fight even harder because being the stupid rascal is even

> more unbearable. The healthy child knows somewhere that he or she will grow up and be an adult; the severely or profoundly handicapped adult will always be dependent.
>
> (Sinason 1992: 227)

One of the questions that the group explored was what sort of independence is possible when you have a disability? The group created a piece of drama called the 'rubbish baby'. This particular drama ended with the discussion circle at the end of the session where one of the members was able to talk about his feelings, particularly how sick he was of being treated like a baby. The 'rubbish baby' bears a truth about this group's experience, which is hard to contemplate. Finding a means to contain such difficult aspects of their experience, I believe, makes it possible for them to go on to name and to state how they feel. I suggest that the quality of the tutor–therapist dialogue played a significant part in enabling the young people to feel safe enough to explore such difficult aspects of their experience. The quality of this dialogue was in turn influenced by the understanding and support gained through dialogue with senior managers.

Is it worth it? The value of dramatherapy within education

Whether it is worth examining our fears, our anxieties, and our inner worlds, and whether this contributes to our well-being and our ability to develop, is central to answering the question, 'Is there a role for dramatherapy in education?' What I saw in the two years of working with this group was development in terms of the ability of the group:

- to take responsibility for the way the sessions were used
- to manage feelings that came up in the sessions
- to empathize with each other and to support each other
- to use language
- to make and sustain relationships
- to do tasks independently
- to conduct themselves with confidence and self-esteem.

All of these abilities were present both in and out of sessions. I am not saying that dramatherapy alone was responsible for all of these things. I am suggesting, however, that the ability of the college and the staff team to create an opportunity for this therapy space and the ability of the tutor and myself to forge a mutually respectful relationship were vital components in promoting such development. My belief is that giving the young people the opportunity to discover a means of exploring and expressing something of their experience of being adolescents with a disability was a powerful impetus to their maturity and development as young people.

Language can quintessentially separate out a piece of experience

My understanding of how dramatherapy was helpful begins with Stern's (1985) ideas about language. He writes about the role of language in terms of representing and sharing our experience. Stern suggests that the relationship between non-verbal experience and that part of it that can be transformed into words can take many forms. In the ideal case, the piece of experience that language separates out is quintessential and captures the whole experience beautifully. He suggests that language is generally thought to function in this ideal way but rarely does. There will be times when the language and the experience to which it refers coexist more or less well. Some parts of the experience may be poorly represented, or may not be represented at all, and will be cut off and have a misnamed or poorly understood existence. There will be areas of experience that cannot readily be given verbal expression. I am suggesting that there were aspects of the experience of these young disabled people that were initially very poorly represented. I am suggesting that one of the tasks of the group was to reclaim, by naming, experience that had been running underground, that had been cut off, misnamed and poorly understood. What made it possible to reclaim and to name some of this experience was the opportunity to play with and gain a perspective on the experience by viewing it and having it viewed.

Alvarez (1992) suggests that what is most important in terms of a person's ability to assimilate ideas is the possibility of gaining perspective. She points out that some people 'may be alerted to a new experience for what seems to be the first time not when it is happening inside of them, but, rather, when it is seen to be happening inside someone else' (1992: 80).

What becomes an important process before ownership of an idea can take place is the opportunity 'to explore it and examine it from a perspective or location that makes it viewable and examinable' (Alvarez 1992: 80).

The way the young people rushed to the sessions and the confidence with which they used the space was testament to the value they placed on the sessions. My sense is that they valued the opportunity to have a space in which they had control. They valued a space where judgement was temporarily suspended. No matter how cruelly, angrily or sadly they represented their experience, it was accepted as a part of their experience that was valid. It needed witnessing and holding.

I would suggest that dramatherapy can have a variety of useful roles to play within education and that the most important role of all is its contribution to the very thinking process itself. Experience can be played with and owned. Ideas can be played with and owned.

Conclusion

For dramatherapy within education to be possible at all and, moreover, to be effective:

- We need to be clear about the dramatherapy on offer and what sort of outcomes can be expected.
- We need to be clear from the outset about the issues and difficulties in creating and maintaining a therapy space, i.e. the need for a room, privacy, continuity, dialogue with staff and a clarity about the relationship between therapy and teaching.
- We need to maintain a dialogue at all levels within the institution.

Acknowledgements

The Editors express grateful thanks to The British Association of Dramatherapists, who kindly granted permission for this extract from the article originally published in *The BADth Journal of Dramatherapy* Vol. 23, No. 1, Spring 2001.

References

Alvarez, A. (1992) *Live Company: Psychoanalytic Psychotherapy with Autistic, Borderline, Deprived and Abused Children*. London: Routledge.
Bion, W.R. (1970) *Attention and Interpretation*. London: Tavistock.
Harris Williams, M. (ed.) (1987) *Collected Papers of Martha Harris and Esther Bick*. Scotland: Clunie Press.
Obholzer, A. and Roberts, V. (eds.) (1994) *The Unconscious at Work. Individual and Organisational Stress in the Human Services*. London: Routledge.
Sinason, V. (1992) *Mental Handicap and the Human Condition: New Approaches from the Tavistock*. London: Free Association Books.
Stern, D.N. (1985) *The Interpersonal World of the Infant*. New York: Basic Books.
Waddell, M. (2002) *Inside Lives*. London: Karnac.

14 Staff sharing: an integrative approach to peer supervision

Catherine Kelly and Talya Bruck

Introduction

Schools are increasingly expected to be able to demonstrate standards of emotional health and wellbeing (e.g. Department for Children, Schools and Families 2008; Department of Health and Department for Education and Science 2005). However, when working with students with special educational needs, teachers report high levels of stress and may describe feelings of anger, frustration, and of 'being at a loss' (Male and May 1997). Furthermore, OFSTED (2004) concluded that teachers in only a third of secondary schools were considered to be effective in meeting the needs of pupils with social, emotional and behavioural difficulties. The value of supporting groups of teachers in schools to manage pupil difficulties has long been established within psychotherapy and educational psychology practice (Chesner 1999; Farouk 2004), and support groups may be considered a particularly effective method of supervision, as school staff can experience professional isolation (Bedward and Daniels 2005), particularly in relation to social, emotional and behavioural difficulties (Miller 2003).

Effective working in groups has been extensively studied in the business and organizational psychology literature (Janz, Colquitt and Noe 1997) and, more recently, is increasingly studied in helping professions (Atkinson, Wilkin, Stott, Doherty and Kinder 2002). However, the literature also suggests that effective work in groups does not occur spontaneously and, furthermore, inherent features of groups can work against efficient communication. This chapter will outline the literature that informed this approach to ensuring effective communication within peer supervision groups of teaching staff. The particular procedure, building on Gill and Monsen's (1996) staff sharing scheme, will then be outlined and consideration given to setting up groups in school. Finally, a brief evaluation of the model will be described.

Peer supervision with groups of teachers

Farouk (2004) details two interacting psycho-social processes that influence the effective functioning of school staff groups: the influence of school culture and/or subgroup culture on group members and their ability to contribute to the group; and the dynamics that occur within the group.

For example, the group facilitator has various group maintenance functions, including 'gate keeping', which involves 'reducing the activity of overactive members and increasing the activity of overtly passive members' (Schein 1988: 52). This is described as 'encouraging everybody to contribute at an early stage and by sensitively asking quieter members of the group to give their opinions' (Farouk 2004: 213). The detail of how a consultant or facilitator influences these internal processes of a group are not detailed, which may be considered surprising given the wealth of literature concerned with group dynamics, including for example how groups take decisions, how groups interact and the roles that individuals adopt for themselves (Allen and Hecht 2004; Hill 1982). Additionally, when discussing pupils with special educational needs, groups have been found to have: a tendency to defer to authority, inequality of contributions, dominance of particular viewpoints, constraints on open debate and a desire to minimize conflict (Cline 1989; Bartolo 2001).

Group problem solving

Abelson and Woodman (1983) concluded that a laissez-faire approach to task and social processes in groups was unlikely to pay dividends and to be effective a group must manage its decision-making process so that the strengths of group decision-making are not lost. What are the barriers to effective problem-solving in groups?

- Inequality of contributions (Cline 1989).
- A tendency to rush to consensus without fully evaluating alternatives (Janis 1982).
- A 'majority wins' rather than 'truth wins' approach (Stasser and Stewart 1992).
- Information not already held in common less likely to be sought (Stasser, Vaughan and Stewart 2000).
- Group brainstorming of ideas is less efficient than individual idea generation (Diehl and Stroebe 1991).

Facilitating problem-solving in groups

Ensuring equality of contributions and using structured problem-solving

Traditional unstructured discussion is often inefficient and it is suggested that performance in groups can be enhanced through structured problem-solving techniques, to facilitate equality of contributions, and exploration of different and possibly divergent or contradictory perspectives (Janis 1982; Rogelberg, Barnes-Farrell and Low 1992; Van de Ven and Delbecq 1974).

Generating ideas

Unstructured idea generation and sharing in groups can be a relatively inefficient process (Paulus and Yang 2000), and freely interacting groups tend to produce fewer ideas than individuals brainstorming alone (Diehl and Stroebe 1991). Productivity loss (in terms of numbers of ideas generated) is not due to less speaking time but having to wait, as participants either forget some of their ideas or generate fewer ideas as they are focused on rehearsal whilst waiting. Paulus (2000) found that structured group interaction followed by individual reflection before decisions are made allows for incubation of ideas, a greater number of ideas generated and better decisions. Given the tendency for school staff groups to rush to solutions before fully considering aspects of the problem (Gill and Monsen 1996), it was felt important to include some individual reflection on the problem as well as a clear problem-solving structure in this model of staff sharing.

Consensus and disagreement

The evidence indicates that group performance can be inhibited by disagreement and tensions among members. Janis (1982) suggests that it is the facilitation of different, divergent or contradictory viewpoints before collectively focusing on workable solutions that is effective in producing superior group outcomes. Tjosvold and Tjosvold (1995) found that disagreement seemed to arouse the participant's motivation to understand other's reasoning, resulting in greater understanding of the other person's perspective. Additionally, a further positive effect of group discussion is the opportunity for verbalization and reiteration of a viewpoint, which may increase an individual's own comprehension, understanding and retention of information (Johnson and Johnson 1989).

The staff sharing procedure

Dramatherapy sessions take place within a basic shape or format, consisting of four sections or elements: *warm up*, in preparation for the work ahead and to create the space; *focusing*, a period of more direct engagement with the content of the work; *closure and de-roling*, marking the end of the main work; and *completion*, creating a space for integration of the material and preparation for leaving (Jones 2007). These elements of a dramatherapy session and ideas from research into group processes regarding equality of contributions, structured problem-solving, generating ideas, and facilitating consensus and disagreement informed the structure and process of this approach. The format of the sessions was as follows:

- Warm-up activity.
- Feedback from previous session.
- Present new issue.
- Clarifying questions.
- Reflective questions.
- Theories/hypotheses.
- Strategies.
- Reflection.

Timescales for each part of the procedure should be discussed and agreed with the group beforehand, according to time given for the session. To maintain and continue developing the group identity and building of trust, a warm-up activity is included each week. This also serves the function of delineating the boundary of the sessions from the 'outside' world of the school. The final reflection activity also acknowledges this boundary. Continuity between sessions is supported by feedback on the issue presented at the previous meeting. This is a brief time for the person who presented previously to say how things have been. It is stressed that it is not expected that all difficulties have been 'solved', but perhaps there has been a small change in the relationship between the teacher and young person and that the dynamic between them has begun to shift.

The next part of the session focuses on a 'new' concern. The case presenter begins talking about the issue uninterrupted for a specific amount of time. While the presenter is talking, one of the facilitators records the main points. Once the presenter is finished, the group may be invited to briefly contribute any additional information. Each person in the group in turn then asks any clarifying questions, i.e. what, how, where and so on. These questions clarify the issue presented and may add further information. Questions are asked in turn in order to facilitate equality of participation (Rogelberg, Barnes-Farrell and Low 1992). The next stage, reflective questioning, is intended to help the staff look at the concern from a new perspective, giving them perhaps a deeper understanding of the young person and their difficulties. The aim is to start to look at the young person in more of a psychodynamic and systemic way. Example questions may include 'when is the problem not so bad?', 'how does it make you feel?', 'what is the young person getting out of this behaviour?' and so on. The ideas of transference, countertransference and projection (Halton 1994) can be introduced, along with some solution-focused questioning. Again, to ensure equality of contributions, the group asks questions in turn.

When the questioning stage is complete, the group moves on to the theories/hypotheses stage. Group members are invited to individually reflect on and record their current view of the problem situation. Ideas are recorded individually as group generation of ideas is less efficient than individual initial generation of ideas (Paulus 2000). Group members' hypotheses regarding the problem are then shared in turn, usually one from each person. Viewpoints are shared following the individual idea generation, as verbalizing a viewpoint and explaining reasoning increases comprehension and retention of that viewpoint (Johnson and Johnson 1989). The presenter can comment in response to each viewpoint in order to facilitate open discussion of opposing views (Tjosvold and Tjosvold 1995).

Next, the group members are asked to consider possible strategies/interventions that would assist the problem from their perspective. These are again recorded individually and then shared in turn. At the end of the session the written hypotheses and strategies, as well as the notes made by the facilitator, are available for the presenter to take away to consider in their own time. This is to allow an opportunity for incubation of the ideas put forward (Paulus 2000).

Setting up groups

Issues for consideration when setting up staff sharing in a school include the contract between the facilitators and the school and the contract between group members at the start of the group and once it is underway. Initial negotiation regarding the work should include the following:

- Aims and objectives of the group.
- Will the group run during staff's own time or during allocated time? (The latter can be more effective as this indicates to the staff how seriously the school are taking the intervention.)
- The length of each session.
- How is the purpose and function of the group described to staff (i.e. it is a facilitated problem solving forum rather than outside agencies giving advice)?
- How many/which staff will attend (i.e. teachers, teachers and teaching assistants, management)?
- The number of sessions.
- What room will be used, will it be the same each week (this is important and aids continuity)?

The first session is usually a training session to introduce the staff sharing procedure and to begin building a group identity through establishing a working contract for the group and engaging in group activities. In order for the group to be effective it is vital that the group feels safe enough to begin the journey together. So, just as within therapy, in order for the client to feel safe enough to explore their issues, it is important to develop an understanding of and agree the contract (Langley 2006).

Writing a group contract together is likely to include, for example: confidentiality, mutual respect, listening and being non-judgemental. The sessions are not intended to directly focus on teachers' own issues but, due to the nature of the procedure and particularly through the reflective questioning, an individual's issues might be raised. The sessions may also examine issues relating to different teaching practices and styles, and some members of staff may feel uncomfortable. It is therefore necessary to help support them in creating a space that is confidential and non-judgemental and that makes them feel safe enough to share relevant issues. 'The client usually knows immediately without explanation that things are possible here which could not be broached elsewhere' (Brazier 2008: 1).

It is key to establish that there is no hierarchy in the group; each group member is just as important as the next, and the group will be relying on everyone's expertise. Also imperative to the running of the group is an agreement that the facilitators are not thought to be the 'experts' as this also sets the group up to possibly feel that what they have to offer is not of value and the facilitators will at the end of the session 'save' the day.

Evaluation

The staff sharing model was carried out in an inner-city one form entry primary school. Seven fortnightly sessions took place and they were evaluated through the use of before and after questionnaires. Responses showed that at the end of the seven sessions the participants all felt better able to both prevent and deal with difficult behaviours. They found dealing with difficult behaviours less stressful. Participants were asked to rate different causes of difficult behaviour in the primary classroom. These were grouped into four categories: teacher actions, pupil vulnerability, adverse family circumstances and strictness in the classroom (see Miller 2003). Following the staff sharing sessions, participants rated teacher actions as slightly more important in causing difficult behaviour than it had been rated before the sessions. There was no change in participants' ratings of pupil vulnerability as a cause of difficult behaviour. There was a slight increase in participants' perceptions of the importance of adverse family circumstances. Participants rated strictness in the classroom as slightly less important than previously.

In response to the question, 'What aspects of the sessions were most useful and why?', all participants made positive comments, including:

- It was great to hear each other in an equal forum.
- Taking ideas from a wide range of staff.
- Sharing ideas concerning children's behaviour.
- Discussing individual children and trying to solve problems.
- Useful to listen to peers.

- Discussing issues and offering strategies.
- It helps to reflect, bounce ideas off each other and listen to new viewpoints.
- Positive sharing of ideas.
- Sharing theories and strategies; this was useful as views and opinions were discussed openly.

Conclusion

Today, the teaching profession is required to have many skills other than subject knowledge and classroom control. They have a duty of care towards each student and each other, which requires them to support emotional health and wellbeing. Creating a forum for teachers to discuss issues of concern that they are not able to address elsewhere is extremely valuable and important. If we are to hold the whole child in mind, should we not be supporting teachers in this way as children spend a large majority of their day in school? This chapter has outlined a staff sharing structure that brings together thinking from dramatherapy and educational psychology to support the teacher in addressing a concern regarding a pupil and to assist teachers in supporting each other through modelling effective group communication.

References

Abelson, M. A. and Woodman, R. W. (1983). 'Review of research on team effectiveness: Implications for teams in schools'. *School Psychology Review*, 12, 125–136.

Allen, N. J. and Hecht, T. D. (2004). 'The romance of teams: Toward an understanding of its psychological underpinnings and implications'. *Journal of Occupational and Organizational Psychology*, 77, 439–461.

Atkinson, M., Wilkin, A., Stott, A., Doherty, P., and Kinder, K. (2002). *Multi-Agency Working: A Detailed Study*. Slough: NFER.

Bartolo, P. A. (2001). 'How disciplinary and institutional orientation influences professionals' decision-making about early childhood disability'. *Educational and Child Psychology*, 18 (2), 88–106.

Bedward, J. and Daniels, H. R. J. (2005). 'Collaborative solutions – clinical supervision and teacher support teams: reducing professional isolation through effective peer support'. *Learning in Health and Social Care*, 4 (2), 53–66.

Brazier, D. D. (2008). 'Amida Trust Papers: Safe Space'. Available from: http://www.amidatrust.com/article_safespace.html (Accessed 10 February 2008).

Chesner, A. (1999). 'Dramatherapy supervision: Historical issues and supervisory settings', in E. Tselikas-Portmann (ed.), *Supervision and Dramatherapy*. London: Kingsley.

Cline, T. (1989). 'Making case conferences more effective: a checklist for monitoring and training'. *Children and Society*, 3 (2), 99–106.

Department for Children, Schools and Families (2008). *Targeted Mental Health in*

Schools Project: Using the evidence to inform your approach: a practical guide to head teachers and commissioners. London: DCSF Publications.

Department of Health and Department for Education and Skills (2005). *National Healthy Schools Status. A Guide for Schools*. London: DH Publications. Available from http://www.wiredfor health.gov.uk/PDF/NHSS_A_Guide_for_Schools_10_05.pdf (Accessed 10 February 2008).

Diehl, M. and Stroebe, W. (1991). 'Productivity loss in idea-generating groups: Tracking down the blocking effect'. *Journal of Personality and Social Psychology*, 61, 392–403.

Farouk, S. (2004). 'Group work in schools: A process consultation approach'. *Educational Psychology in Practice*, 20 (3), 207–220.

Gill, D. and Monsen, J. (1996). 'The staff sharing scheme: a school-based management system for working with challenging child behaviour'. *Educational and Child Psychology*, 12 (2), 71–79.

Halton, W. (1994). 'Some unconscious aspects of organizational life – contributions from psychoanalysis', in A. Obholzer and V. Z. Robergs (eds.), *The Unconscious at Work*. New York: Routledge.

Hill, G. W. (1982). 'Group versus individual performance: Are N + 1 heads better than one'? *Psychological Bulletin*, 91, 517–539.

Janis, I. L. (1982). *Groupthink*, 2nd edition. Boston: Houghton Mifflin.

Janz, B. D., Colquitt, J. A., and Noe, R. A. (1997). 'Knowledge worker team effectiveness: the role of autonomy, interdependence, team development and contextual support variables'. *Personnel Psychology*, 50, 877–904.

Johnson, D. W. and Johnson, R. T. (1989). *Cooperation and Competition: Theory and Research*. Edina, MN: Interaction Book Company.

Jones, P. (2007). *Drama as Therapy: Theory, Practice and Research*. London: Routledge.

Langley, D. (2006). *An Introduction to Dramatherapy*, Thousand Oaks, CA: Sage.

Male, D. B. and May, D. S. (1997). 'Stress, burnout and workload in teachers of children with special educational needs'. *British Journal of Special Education*, 24 (3), 133–140.

Miller, A. (2003). *Teachers, Parents and Classroom Behaviour. A Psychosocial Approach*. Milton Keynes: Open University Press.

OFSTED (2004). *Special Educational Needs and Disability: Towards Inclusive Schools*. London: OFSTED.

Paulus, P. B. (2000). 'Groups, teams and creativity: The creative potential of idea generating groups'. *Applied Psychology: An International Review*, 49, 237–262.

Paulus, P. B. and Yang, H. C. (2000). 'Idea generation in groups: A basis for creativity in organizations'. *Organizational Behavior and Human Decision Processes*, 82, 76–87.

Rogelberg, S. G., Barnes-Farrell, J. L., and Lowe, C. A. (1992). 'The step-ladder technique: An alternative group structure facilitating effective group decision making'. *Journal of Applied Psychology*, 77 (5), 730–737.

Schein, H. E. (1988). *Process Consultation: Its Role in Organization Development*, 2nd edn., Vol. 1. Wokingham: Addison-Wesley.

Stasser, G. and Stewart, D. (1992). 'Discovery of hidden profiles by decision-making groups: Solving a problem versus making a judgement'. *Journal of Personality and Social Psychology*, 63 (3), 426–434.

Stasser, G., Vaughan, S. I., and Stewart, D. D. (2000). 'Pooling unshared information: The benefits of knowing how access to information is distributed among members'. *Organizational Behavior and Human Decision Processes*, 82, 102–116.

Tjosvold, D. and Tjosvold, M. M. (1995). 'Cooperation theory, constructive controversy and effectiveness: Learning from crises', in R. A. Guzzo and E. Salas (eds.), *Team Effectiveness and Decision Making in Organizations*, 333–381. San Francisco: Jossey-Bass.

Van de Ven, A. H. and Delbecq, A. L. (1974). 'The effectiveness of nominal, Delphi and interacting group decision-making processes'. *Academy of Management Journal*, 17 (4), 605–621.

15 'I'm not so sure, Miss'. The concept of uncertainty and dramatherapy practice within the context of transdisciplinary work in an educational setting

Daniel Mercieca

Introduction

In this chapter I wish to share how the 'not-knowing' (Anderson and Goolishian 1992) stance in narrative therapies has influenced my practice as a dramatherapist within a residential and educational set-up. Knowing about not knowing has allowed a fostering of newness within me as a dramatherapist working in a context where knowing the right answers is considered as important. This 'newness' has influenced the work with the clients I meet, mostly male latency-aged children, adolescents and their families.

I will be writing about the use of the art object/expression in promoting a stance of 'safe uncertainty' (Mason 1993) in the therapist, the clients and other professionals within the context of a trans-disciplinary support services team within an educational and residential set-up. I will also be considering how this stance can be extended in working with the different systems around the child.

I work with children and adolescents who face traumatic experiences or relational difficulties within their immediate family and may require an out of home placement and/or a specialized kind of educational placement. The educational setting I work within focuses on each individual student by assessing his learning needs and developing an individual plan that utilizes small group and non-formal learning opportunities. Within an overall set-up that values a preventive and relational approach to education, individual plans may include a variety of therapeutic interventions alongside other more educationally oriented provisions.

The set-up also includes a residential service that provides various types of out of home care placements to meet the needs of children and adolescents who are not able to live within their family of origin. Out of home care may be a temporary provision with the ultimate aim being that of family restoration or a more permanent placement. As a dramatherapist, I coordinate a trans-disciplinary therapeutic team that provides therapeutic and assessment interventions to a number of clients and their families. The trans-disciplinary therapeutic team includes the services of a family therapist, an educational psychologist, a Gestalt psychotherapist and a counselling psychologist alongside the dramatherapy service. This sets the context for a most fertile exchange between disciplines.

Over a period of ten years, the dramatherapy service has evolved from one focusing on the individual child to one that, whilst holding the individual child's needs in focus, views the child and works with the child in the various meaning exchanges within which the child participates. This may constitute working with teachers, care workers, family members, foster carers, family therapists, prospective adoptive parents, social workers and siblings in care in other out of home settings. Such a shift has been complemented by the setting up of the aforementioned therapeutic team.

Within this shift, whilst still acknowledging the need for a distinction between the educational/learning space and the therapeutic one, I would strive not to be organized by such a distinction. I became more aware of how a very rigid distinction could limit me in terms of working with the whole system. The therapeutic, set apart space needed to be respected yet at the same time it ran the risk of developing into a hermitage. As I learnt to trust positions of uncertainty, I could start appreciating the therapy within education and the learning within therapy. It is paradoxical at times that in our efforts to heal the whole person we carefully segment and dissect this oneness into parts that each profession claims that it can manage. Yet within this dissection the sum of these parts hardly ever adds up to the energy that pertains to the whole child.

First vignette

I am witnessing Alan, a 12-year-old, working with a number of pebbles to represent his family. I am seeing the way the family members, represented by different pebbles on a solid square surface, are all assembled around the predicament that he presents in therapy. Alan suffers from a medical condition that has impinged on his life in such a way that he has been close to dying and required an innumerable number of medical interventions since birth. At present he needs to self-administer a medical treatment every few hours and his parents and sibling are concerned that he is not administering this as frequently as he should. During the pebble manipulation, my interventions are intended as moving with him from one step behind, asking questions that promote clarification and curiosity. I am trying to take a position of a 'naive enquirer' (Bannister 1998), having faith that this activity will reveal surprises to us but at the same time containing my doubt that perhaps it won't.

The family (two parents and an older sister) are invited to the session and the boy wants them to witness his art object, i.e. the assembly of pebbles. Before this witnessing, within a verbal check-in space that precedes the actual action-based intervention, words were exchanged but the positions appeared rather fixed and limiting. Whilst useful in terms of empowering all to clarify the aims of why we were meeting, these conversations seemed to put the child in the position of the problem bearer who needed to change.

As the family starts witnessing the assembly of pebbles, space is opened up for exploration. Now the surface with the stones on it, our mini stage, becomes the focus of attention as Alan explains his creation. His family members are asking questions. The father refers to the dark larger pebble representing the medical problem. As he grabs this pebble he wonders why it seems to be so difficult for his son to just take hold and get rid of it, out of the playing surface and out of the family. He wonders why this seems to be so tough. Alan explains that such an act is not possible. He is aware that the medical problem is there and will remain. He explains that when he tries to think about it not being there, that actually makes him not take care of himself and hence not self-medicate. Administering the self-medication is a reminder of the medical difficulties' presence. The mother is very emotional and comments on how this statement is new to her and how she never thought her son could reflect so deeply on his situation. Then we proceed to experiment with how the stones could be in a different position. As we play around with new positions, Alan comments on how he feels family members closer to him at this point.

As we worked over a number of weeks, the child, the family as witnesses, and I could see how the problem could be moved. The dark stone started being more amenable to being shifted . . . not thrown away. We could see how the family could take a different assembly. At a point, Alan commented how the stone was obstructing his view of the family and the support he could receive from them. Mum commented how the dark stone seemed to shadow and restrict her view of her son. Once Alan moved the dark stone to the side lines, now parents and child were facing each other. Even in our pre-activity talking space, new adolescent boundary-setting difficulties tended to be considered. We weren't just speaking about the medical problem. Paradoxically Alan welcomed this new introduction as evidence that he 'fits in' with his friends and the general youth culture.

During future sessions, as he manipulated the pebbles, Alan became aware how the problem pebble seems to function as that which kept him glued to his mum and near other members of his family. He became aware of the following pattern. As long as he has a problem, they will worry about him. As long as they worry about him, they will be around him; almost a sort of guarantee that he will remain the 'special child'. The whole family seemed to be conditioned by the patterns that emerged out of their constructions around 'the special child'.

Within this piece of work, rather than verbalizing my interpretation of the art object as an expression of the unconscious, I saw my role as that of allowing the client and the family to come to their own interpretation of the art object . . . to come to different interpretations . . . to witness the expression as fluid and 'could be moved'. I tried to operate from a position of 'not knowing' (Anderson and Goolishian 1992) or rather of being aware of my knowing but not letting it condition me down one path.

The 'not-knowing' stance

Anderson explains this position as a position where 'the therapist's pre-experience and pre-knowledge do not lead' (1993: 325). The approach is rooted in contemporary hermeneutics, and social constructionism. In the hermeneutical view there is no privileged position from where to perceive and describe experience because this view advocates for the consideration of a multiplicity of positions. Anderson and Goolishian (1992) see the 'not knowing' approach as one based on an acknowledgment of human systems as language- and meaning-generating systems rather than something finite whose workings and laws of construction need to be understood. This position is to be located within the narrative therapies (Andersen 1991; Anderson and Goolishian 1988; Parry 1991; Penn and Frankfurt 1994; White and Epston 1990). As Rober (1999) explains, narrative therapies are therapeutic models that use conversation, stories, dialogues, narrative and text as the dominant metaphor in the therapeutic exchange.

Within the hermeneutical view, in contrast with systemic cybernetics, the system does not create a problem. Within contemporary hermeneutics and social constructionism, the perspective adopted is that languaging about problems gives rise to systems.

> . . . problems and the systems organized by them are not fixed entities existing over time until they are resolved or repaired. Problems and problem-organizing systems are changed and reinterpreted just as often, and just as rapidly, as the other narratives around which we organize meaning and social exchange.
>
> (Anderson and Goolishian 1988: 8)

Whilst the challenging behaviour of a child who faces emotional and behavioural difficulties is a problem in the school yard, isn't the way that child is spoken about in the staff room and amongst his peers also problematic? How does the language we use and live in within our schools colour our actions? Can we really differentiate between what we say about children and what we do with them?

It is within this social constructionist perspective that the not knowing approach needs to be framed. It is an approach that privileges the transformational power of narrative as a dialogic exchange, within the understanding that events or lives can be re-related and that within that re-relation, new and different meaning will be generated.

A most valid elaboration of this model or perspective is Mason's (1993) exploration of a position of 'safe uncertainty'. Mason tries to bridge the gap between uncertainty and expertise through such concepts as 'authoritative doubt' (1993). He presents not knowing as a stance of resisting to understand too quickly. Quoting Krull, he argues that 'it is still possible to have strong beliefs and still be consistent with a stance of not knowing' (Krull 1988, cited in Mason 1993: 191). He contrasts this position with positions of safe certainty, unsafe certainty and unsafe uncertainty, whilst presenting it as one where 'new explanations can be placed alongside rather than instead of, in competition with, the explanations that clients and therapists bring' (Mason 1993: 194).

The 'not-knowing' stance and the art object

One can approach the exploration of the art object/expression through a not-knowing stance. As Levy comments, the tendency amongst psychodynamic approaches has been to move away from sole reliance on interpretation in using play techniques in therapeutic work with children. He asserts that 'child therapists . . . must be more comfortable with ambiguity in their encounters with their clients' (2008: 284).

In contrast to an interpretative knowing stance, the creative act, its expression and eventual exploration can become a rich source of transformation as new meaning can be created.

> The therapist's role, expertise and emphasis is to develop a free conversational space and to facilitate an emerging dialogical process in which this 'newness' can occur. The emphasis is not to produce change but to open space for conversation. In this hermeneutic view, change in therapy is represented by the dialogical creation of new meaning.
>
> (Anderson and Goolishian 1992: 29)

Within dramatherapy, new meaning is most likely to be generated if we manage to approach the creative act, be it a self-elicited story, a constellation of small objects or a role play, through a sense of 'genuine curiosity' (Anderson and Goolishian 1992: 29). Thus through such a verbal or nonverbal exploration of the creative act we would be allowing the 'not yet said stories' and the 'not yet taken positions' to be said and taken.

Second Vignette: of buoys and boys

During a dramatherapy session, John is flicking through some photos in order to choose some to represent how he feels at present. He is used to this ritual in order to communicate his current needs and feelings. John lives in residential care due to the fact that his father is unknown and his mum faces a lot of inconsistency in taking care of him. Before the session his social worker informs me that his mum has left the country again to join a partner in another country. His social worker comments that John has never spoken about this with her, even though the adolescent knows about mum and about the fact that his social worker knows as well. Teachers are quite perplexed about the fact that though he is very promising, he seems to lose his grounding in class and finds it very difficult to concentrate or stay on task.

He chooses a photo of a buoy at sea. He is not sure what it means to him but despite his need to hide his face from me, he manages to communicate his interest in this photo. I am curious about the possibilities. The photo may be explored and so I invite John to create a story about this buoy. John takes up my invitation. He creates a story about how this buoy once lived near another buoy. Both buoys were attached to their own large boulders under the sea, yet the little buoy's rope was not so strong, at least not as strong as the other buoy's rope. Eventually, in a storm, the small buoy's rope was torn, and this buoy was carried by the sea current, unable to decide its own fate. It had to face the open seas, the ever-changing current, the waves and the weather on it own, without its own boulder. Yet, eventually, the small buoy found out that somehow it could swim, it could make an effort to move against the current and make its own choices regarding how to find help. The little buoy searched for help. It managed to find a substitute other buoy to which to attach its dangling rope.

We proceeded to enact this part of the story. Whilst in the role of the little buoy, John tells me that whilst he feels safe hanging on to the substitute buoy, he (as the little buoy) is still concerned about trying to get help to reach the 'missing' buoy again. In fact he chooses to end the story with the little buoy finding the 'missing buoy' once again. Yet, he commented that this story is not finished, because the small buoy still needs to attach its dangling rope to somewhere safe.

Whilst the connection to external life in the above metaphor may be evident, my task was that of enabling an exploration of the story through enactment, and opening conversations about it, whilst staying within the roles created and the enactment space. As we worked, new stories emerged regarding the unpredictability of the weather, regarding how in this particular world it seems that, contrary to custom, the small buoys have to look out for the bigger ones. Other stories emphasized resilience and highlighted the small buoy's determination and how it wanted to live and seek good waters to live in.

Yet, exploring these stories and reaching emotional catharsis through working within the metaphor through a not-knowing stance, is only one aspect of the therapeutic intervention.

In discussing the use of play techniques in understanding disturbed behaviour in schools, Mawson states that

> neither analytic understanding of the child from a limited contact, nor discussion with those in caretaking or parental roles, is sufficient in itself, but rather . . . the combination needs to be made in the service of containing staff anxieties evoked by the child.
>
> (1986: 53)

In the approach being presented within this chapter the 'analytic understanding of the child' in the above quote is being reframed as 'the collaborative understanding with the child'. This understanding needs to be linked with the other persons who are caring for him.

During future sessions, John asked whether he could tell the story to his social worker. The conversational space was opened up as the residential social worker aided our exploration. The conversation shifted onto how there could be different endings to the same story. We explored how, maybe, the small buoy would need its own grounding so that it would not be totally dependent on the larger buoy. John warned us how bad weather could strike again and shift buoys around once again. Now within the confines and safety of the metaphor, the social worker could be in a space where together with John they could contain this story.

What stayed with me in this particular work is how the child and the social worker were able to juggle with the story, to explore new meaning, to create new meaning around the experience. Whilst it is tempting to proceed along one direction and softly get the client to follow, the stance of 'not knowing' allows for the co-presence of new narratives; the 'not yet said' (Anderson and Goolishian, 1988). The social worker was also able to view the child in a different way as new meaning was being generated.

The 'not yet said'

Through the use of the metaphor, the 'not yet said' may find the space to be said in the form of stories that may stand out as alternatives to the dominant stories in a family's life (White and Epston 1990). Gadamer (1975), citing Hans Lipps' circle of the unexpressed, refers to this as the 'infinity of the unsaid'.

As a trans-disciplinary team, this possibility of working with the infinity of the unsaid has been important, especially when working with a residential and educational set-up that at times is tightly organized by the trauma that the children and their families bring (Bentovim 1995). As Bentovim maintains,

> the effect of trauma associated with secrecy and silence organizes family members into action systems which are self-maintaining, organizing the family and those professionals who come into contact with the family.
>
> (1995: 119)

Thus, allowing the untold stories to be expressed through creative expression becomes even more important in order to allow staff and family members to enter a space where the un-talkable can be talked about and juggled around.

At times, in a specialized educational setting the formal story of the child, mostly speaking about abuse and trauma, stands in front of us as some sort of megalith. It is so tempting to cling onto one interpretation even as a reaction to the chaos that needs to be tolerated in particularly stressful moments. There are some enriching models, such as the attachment model or Kohut's (1984) developmental consideration of unmet self–object needs that allow the therapist or educator to feel some sort of safe grounding. Yet a blind reliance on any model may limit our flexibility. We may risk getting stuck in viewing the child as a somewhat static byproduct of a neglectful process. This static perception may lead the staff working with the child into a cycle of helplessness, frequently replaying the dynamics within the child's life, thus the trauma-organized system.

It is important not to disregard the frameworks of such models, yet it is equally important for the therapist to be able to juggle the models around in an inner conversation (Rober 1999) and invite others into this juggling act. It is in the in-between space of internal juggling that one can see the child and his family as meaning-making persons. The challenge is how to invite other persons working with the child into this act of juggling and to tolerate the healthy uncertainty that it provokes.

As Andersen (1993) explains, we are working with nuances in words and expressions that contribute to shifts in descriptions and understanding. As in the first vignette, we are considering the nuances of difference between different family members' comments on the same art object that create the difference and open up space for change. 'In using alternative means of communication, families can begin to engage in a different way, adding an element of surprise to a potentially difficult endeavour' (Manicom and Boronska 2003: 217).

Implications for the role of the therapist and limitations of the approach

As a dramatherapist, adhering to a position of 'safe uncertainty' (Mason 1993) allows me to practise from a position that neither negates taking a stand nor abdicates professional responsibility. It is a decision about not taking one stand and still remaining safe. Where does this safety come from? For me this comes from an acknowledgment that I cannot not influence. As Strong maintains, 'if we cannot avoid influence, to what end do we exercise it in therapy?' (2000: 146). This is an essential question that allows me to reflect on my values, my story, the cultural divide between my values and the values of families who require the services of residential placement, the dominant discourses in my life and how my role as a dramatherapist is socially constructed. These categories need to find their space in my inner conversation, whilst simultaneously attending and participating to the external exchange with clients. They also need to find their space in the conversations that I carry out with parents, teachers and others involved in the child's life.

What further contributes to developing safety is the contribution of the other therapists on the team and other professionals within the educational and residential care set-up. Within an overall context of trust and safety we are learning to cultivate an 'ever-present sensitivity to misunderstandings' (Strong 2000: 146) where differences and divergences become creative possibilities. Yet we still find this very challenging, especially during moments of heightened anxiety and extremely challenging behaviour within the school. When working with a client who has been abusive to others and is being threatened with exclusion, I tend to see the options narrowing. We have experienced difficulty in remaining creative and 'not knowing' within these constraints.

Conclusion

Within the therapeutic idiom presented in this chapter, the dramatherapist takes on the role of an artist allowing for the emergence of newness whilst upholding an ever-present awareness to how the clients and the system are reacting to the 'newness' of the creative process. 'Those who do not know what to do, need something different (unusual) but this something should not be too different (unusual)' (Andersen 1992: 59). This calls for sensitivity towards issues of cultural differences regarding how an individual, a fellow professional, a group of teachers or a family react to the creative therapeutic space. This sensitivity contributes to the safety within a safe uncertain stance. As artists and therapists, we are called to hold a space that allows some 'room for the familiar' (Andersen 1992) where persons may feel safe enough and held enough to allow themselves to be surprised by that which is not there yet! We can hardly claim to want to explore that which is not there yet, be it in education or in therapy, if we decide to remain only faithful to that which we know and which we cherish. Yet what we know and what we cherish needs to be voiced and respected: it provides the safe ground from where we may dare to risk.

Hopefully, through our creative dramatherapists' practice in schools, we can cultivate attitudes that seek not to be limited by that which all of us claim to know. This may lead us and the persons we work with to be curious about how our knowing impacts our listening, our witnessing and our action as we seek to question our finiteness, our prejudices, our local knowledge, our creative potential, our much cherished models and our stories, whilst willing to be surprised. So, I'm not so sure, Miss . . . because I'm willing to find out!

Bibliography

Andersen, T. (1991) *The Reflecting Team: Dialogues and Dialogues About the Dialogues*. New York, W.W. Norton.

Andersen, T. (1992) Reflections on reflecting with families. In S. McNamee and K.J. Gergen (eds.), *Therapy as Social Construction*, 54–67. London, Sage Publications.

Andersen, T. (1993) See and hear, and be seen and heard in reflexive conversations. In S. Friedman (ed.), *The New Language of Change: Constructive Collaboration in Psychotherapy*, 303–321. New York, Guildford.

Anderson, H. (1993) On a roller coaster: A collaborative language systems approach to therapy. In S. Friedman (ed.), *The New Language of Change: Constructive Collaboration in Psychotherapy*, 323–343. New York, Guildford.

Anderson, H. (1997) *Conversation, Language and Possibilities*. New York, Basic Books.

Anderson, H. and Goolishian, H.A. (1988) Human systems as linguistic systems: Preliminary and evolving ideas about the implications for clinical theory. *Family Process*, 27, 371–394.

Anderson, H. and Goolishian, H.A. (1992) The client is the expert: A not-knowing approach to therapy. In S. McNamee and K.J. Gergen (eds.), *Therapy as Social Construction*, 12–21. London, Sage Publications.

Arad, D. (2004) If your mother were an animal, what animal would she be? Creating play stories in family therapy. *Family Process* 43(2), 249–264.

Bannister, A. (2003) *Creative Therapies with Traumatised Children*. London, Jessica Kingsley Publishers.

Bateson, G. (1972) *Steps to an Ecology of the Mind*. New York, Ballantine.

Bentovim, A. (1995) *Trauma-Organized Systems: physical and sexual abuse in families*. London, Karnac Books.

Boal, A. (1995) *The Rainbow of Desire: The Boal Method of Theatre and Therapy*. London, Routledge.

Burr, V. (1995) *An Introduction to Social Constructionism*. London, Routledge.

Cecchin, G. (1987) Hypothesizing, circularity and neutrality revisited: An invitation to curiosity. *Family Process*, 26(4), 405–413.

Churven, P. (2000) A critique of 'collaborative influence': Is there a role for expertise? *Australian and New Zealand Journal of Family Therapy*, 21(3), 150–151.

Dockar-Drysdale, D. (1991) *The Provision of Primary Experience: Winnicottian Work with Children and Adolescents*. London, Jason Aronson.

Gadamer, H. (1975) *Truth and Method*. New York, Continuum.

Gill, E. (1994) *Play in Family Therapy*. New York, The Guildford Press.

Hoffman, L. (1993) *Exchanging Voices: A Collaborative Approach to Family Therapy*. London, Karnac Books.

Jennings, S. (1992) *Dramatherapy with Families, Groups and Individuals: Waiting in the Wings*. London, Jessica Kingsley.

Kohut, H. (1984) *How Does Analysis Cure?* Chicago, University of Chicago Press.

Levy, A.J. (2008) The therapeutic action of play in the psychodynamic treatment of children: a critical analysis. *Clinical Social Work Journal*, 36, 281–291.

Manicom, H. and Boronska, T. (2003) Co-creating change within a child protection system: Integrating art therapy with family therapy practice. *Journal of Family Therapy*, 25(3), 217–232.

Mason, B. (1993) Towards positions of safe uncertainty. *Humans Systems: The Journal of Systemic Consultation & Management*, 4, 189–200.

Mawson, C. (1986) The use of play technique in understanding disturbed behaviour in school. *Psychoanalytic Psychotherapy*, 2(1), 53–61.

Parry, A. (1991) A universe of stories. *Family Process*, 30(1), 37–54.

Pearce, W.B. and Pearce, K.A. (1998) Transcendent storytelling: Abilities for systemic practitioners and their clients. *Human Systems: The Journal of Systemic Consultation & Management*, 9, 3–10.

Penn, P. and Frankfurt, M. (1994) Creating a participant text: Writing, multiple voices, narrative multiplicity. *Family Process*, 33(3), 217–231.

Rober, P. (1999) The therapist's inner conversation in family therapy practice: Some ideas about the self of the therapist, therapeutic impasse, and the process of reflection. *Family Process*, 38(2), 209–221.

Strong, T. (2000) Collaborative influence. *Australian and New Zealand Journal of Family Therapy*, 21(3), 144–150.

White, M. and Epston, D. (1990) *Narrative Means to Therapeutic Ends*. New York, W.W. Norton & Company Inc.

Woodcock, J. (2003) Comment – art therapy and family therapy. *Journal of Family Therapy*, 25(3), 233–235.

16 Self-harm and safeguarding issues in the school and classroom: a partnership approach

Matthew Trustman

> The following are the principal factors associated with increased risk of self-harm among children and adolescents: mental health or behavioural issues, such as depression, severe anxiety and impulsivity; a history of self-harm; experience of an abusive home life; poor communication with parents; living in care or secure institutions.
>
> (SCIE 2005)

'We have the highest rate of self-harm in Europe, but the universal misunderstanding about self-harm is so overwhelming that numbers will rise even further unless we act immediately,' said Catherine McLoughlin, chairwoman of the first ever national inquiry into self-harm among young people. She said that some reports suggested up to one in five adolescents were 'engaging in this self-destructive behaviour', a subject that was surrounded in 'guilt and secrecy'. (*Sunday Observer* 26 March 2006, article on Mental Health Foundation (2006) Truth hurts; report of the national inquiry into self-harm among young people, Mental Health Foundation and Camelot Foundation, London)

Introduction

'Spare Me The Cutter' is a short film I made exploring relationships surrounding a secondary school-aged self-harming girl. This chapter offers some insight into what happened during a recent Personal, Social and Health Education class in a mixed secondary school where the film was shown. In so doing, this chapter explores two themes that emerge from working as a dramatherapist within the relational landscape of a secondary school. The first theme explores the dramatherapist working alongside a teacher and learning support assistant in a Personal, Social and Health Education lesson, in which a session on self-harming is being run; the second points towards the contribution towards safeguarding children from a dramatherapist's understanding of embodiment.

Deliberate self-harm confronts all of us working in education with our own uncertainties and fears about a subject that is difficult to understand, hard to explain, and offers sometimes limited scope for the provision of straightforward answers to concerned teachers and parents. Section One of the Children Act 1989 relates to safeguarding in schools, stating that the welfare of the child is paramount. It requires schools to ensure that appropriate policies and procedures are in place.

In the day-to-day life of those working in schools, it is the spirit of that law and safeguarding children that is reflected in daily teaching practice and school life. Nevertheless, it is not always easy to provide answers to teachers who are concerned to address some of the sensitive issues of mental and emotional health within the classroom. The school environment remains, in the author's view, the best place to begin to address the scarcity of understanding and awareness of the issues involved in self-harming. This chapter considers an approach, drawing on dramatherapy, that is educational, respectful of the diversity of views and backgrounds within classrooms, and that is within the skill sets expected of those working in schools.

Background

There is no one single behaviour associated with deliberate self-harming, and neither is there a single cause or solution; indeed the term 'self-harm' or 'deliberate self-harm' itself is arguably an inappropriate term to use.

The range of behaviours associated with deliberate self-harm are considerable, and popular confusion that exists surrounding deliberate self-harm towards its relationship to attempted suicide compounds the fear and uncertainty surrounding self-harming, and how it might be addressed in schools. It is indeed a very sensitive subject, and it is very important that we look at this in today's world for our children and young people. Although the term deliberate self-harm has been increasingly represented as behaviour that involves wounding, cutting and burning, it is also used in connection with behaviours ranging from drug and alcohol misuse to eating disorders. Recent research (Best 2006) suggested that while teachers working in such locations as Pupil Referral Units are likely to have some knowledge and awareness of self-harm, awareness amongst teachers in mainstream schools remains limited.

Confidence within schools to include lessons on mental health as part of the curriculum appears to be growing. Recent reviews of mental health teaching initiatives (Naylor et al. 2009; Kidger et al. 2009) report on positive outcomes demonstrated by shifts in attitudes and behaviours of pupils having taken part in lessons addressing mental health issues. The extent to which such shifts in awareness and behaviours within these lessons are influenced by the relational environment within the classroom may understandably be a pedagogic concern for teachers. Of equal concern to dramatherapists involved in classroom work, addressing themes of potentially high sensitivity, are issues of safety, boundaries, and disclosure.

The dramatherapist in education offers a unique contribution to the relational landscape of the school that is not confined to the physical limits of the 'therapeutic space' of clinical practice but is equally effective entering into the social poetics of the classroom and the dynamics of teacher–pupil interaction. 'Social poetics' refers here to the process of the emergence of professional practice that arises in respect to the specific environment of the school. This environment is both the explicit physical, political and educational environment and the less visible uncertain and tacit 'site-specific' environment of human relationships and histories, feeling, senses, rumours and hunches that are present within a classroom and the school. In this context the resources of the dramatherapist contribute a useful source of tacit knowledge, method and process available to establish a 'good enough' facilitative environment, one conducive to exploring mental health issues safely and effectively within a classroom setting. The dramatherapist understanding through their work the transformational potential of enabling a safe space can then enter with the teacher and students into a creative, cooperative learning environment seeking understanding and awareness of the complex issues of self-harm.

The dramatherapist in the school

The dramatherapist's engagement in the social poetics of the school extends across several distinct relational spaces within the physical space of the school, amongst school employees, staff and pupils, and will often extend beyond the physical space of the school into the family, social and health services and community local to the school. The dramatherapist is by virtue of the work they do uniquely positioned within the relational networks of a school. Drawing from this network, 'safeguarding' as a daily practice may usefully be considered as a holistic place-sensitive process in which the dramatherapist's contribution plays a significant role.

'Place', as Lippard (1997: 7) reminds us, refers to an evolving, living site of rich emotional and psychological detail, 'A layered location replete with human histories and memories, place has width as well as depth. It is about connections, what surrounds it, what formed it, what happened there, what will happen there'. Lippard, a writer, activist, and curator goes on to explore the 'labyrinthine diversity of personal geography and lived experience' (1997: 5) of local landscape. Engaging with this lived experience involves the therapist in a daily dialogue with the environment that surrounds their clients, a dialogue that invites the engagement of the therapist's intellectual, emotional and sensory resources. Recognizing such sensory experience as a significant source of knowledge draws from approaches to anthropology and ethnographic research that 'advocates the importance of the senses for understanding the way people interact with others and their surroundings' (Howes 2003: 54). This embodied engagement, in the often messy confusion of everyday life, provides the essential backdrop for the dramatherapist to draw on when working with the sense of place encountered in working with clients.

For dramatherapists, this heuristic approach, which recognizes the 'exploratory' and the 'uncertainty' in the practice of 'safeguarding', can provide an additional rich and dynamic resource to draw on to support the safeguarding of young people in their school.

The dramatherapist in the classroom

A group of 25 boys and girls came into their final Citizenship lesson with their current teacher before they moved on to explore issues of sexual behaviour and recreational drugs the following week with their new teacher. The class already knew the theme of the lesson, and there was a regular level of noise and conversation mixed with some excitement at the presence in the room of a new face.

Amongst the class I recognized a few of the faces, and some of them knew me, although no one from this group had been referred to me for dramatherapy. Had there been, the issue of boundaries would have been thought through carefully before committing to work with the class. The school serves families from often challenging social and economic environments and it is sympathetic to the benefits of counselling and dramatherapy. Some 50 nationalities are represented amongst its pupils, with a relatively high percentage of children eligible for free school meals, and on the Special Needs register. It is also a school that, in recent years, has achieved good GCSE results and opened its own sixth form. The school is oversubscribed for the Year 7 intake.

Working as a part-time dramatherapist, I come into the school once a week. In a week the school will have gone through incidents and changes that will influence the course of my work on that day. As I enter the car park I begin to pick up on the mood and atmosphere of the school when greeting the security and other staff, and begin to orient myself towards the day ahead in the school. Distinct rhythms, patterns of movement and sounds fill corridors and social spaces in the playground and school building, an indication of the emotional mood and sentiment of the school on that day, helping me prepare to enter the classroom.

Once the class began to settle I introduced the themes of the lesson. The subject of 'mental health' inevitably, and perhaps healthily, provoked laughter, finger pointing, and nudging amongst some of the class. Others became quiet, while others, I suspect, didn't hear or weren't listening.

In my practice in the class room I seek to acknowledge the range of responses from the young people, working wherever possible to incorporate and validate, by eye contact and words and gestures the wide range of responses that emerge, concerned also to protect and validate those whose responses are less visible or vocal. I provided an overview of some age- and gender-related statistics on issues connected to self-harming, and talked briefly about attempted suicide, types of self-harming and the focus of the short film they were about to see. We talked about the sensitivity of the subject, and that amongst a group of 25 it is very likely that several will know people with mental health illnesses. The group were told that their teacher and myself would be available after the session should anyone want to talk about issues raised by the film.

The film 'Spare Me The Cutter' explores a series of relationships surrounding a young girl who self-harms. The girl, in contrast to the other characters, is not heard and she is shown only in an abstract collage of shots. This is a deliberate device to seek to negate objectifying the victim or positioning the audience in a voyeuristic relationship to her. The characters speak directly to the audience and the pace, music and visual texture of the video seek to draw the audience's attention towards the characters and their commentary on attitudes towards the self-harmer that the film seeks to highlight. When devising the film it was important to consider how this medium could create an audience, rather than a class, with all that that implies for the acts of meaning-making, identification, distancing and engagement between a performance and its audience. Additionally and importantly, the film has now provided a space within the classroom dynamic for the therapist to act as group facilitator, and to invite pupils, after a second showing of the film, to take up the roles of the characters in the film to answer comments offered by the audience. I have learnt that to show the film a second time seems to extend significantly the relationship between the audience and film.

As the film ends, I set up four chairs and invite the pupils to take up the names of the characters and respond, again in character, to the comments made by the audience. With little reluctance the offer is generally accepted. I am always surprised by the speed at which the pupils adopt the roles and by the debate that takes place. On this occasion, I invited a learning support assistant, who was present throughout, to record a paragraph of her reflections. Her comments follow:

> This film provoked reactions that varied from sympathy and understanding for the young girl who was self-harming, to anger and frustration at the way she was perceived by others around her. The students reacted to the mother negatively, focusing on the pressure she put upon her daughter and her anxiety about what friends and neighbours would think. They viewed the father more kindly, but were aware of his distance to the girl and to his own wife. The school mentor was a more ambiguous character. Students argued about how well she had looked after the girl and questioned how much responsibility and authority, in reality, did she have to protect the young girl? They raised questions about who was it in the school who thought it fair to give such responsibility to a girl little more than the age of the girl herself.

The general view was that the family did not communicate sufficiently, the father wanted to give his daughter more space and back off, the mother thought he shouldn't have been involved at all – they both viewed their child's situation in terms of their own feelings, they didn't seem open to know how they might explore how to help their daughter. 'If they couldn't get their marriage right, how could they properly care for their child?'

Responses were thoughtful, articulate and mature for the age group. The whole class seemed involved. Certainly the opportunity to role play the characters in the film and to ask relevant questions provided lively reactions.

One pupil, when confronted by the 'parents' who said that they couldn't handle their daughter's illness, said passionately 'But you can never give up. That's the role of a parent. You never stop trying.'

The session ended with me de-roleing the participants, inviting them to comment on their experience before they rejoined their class and entered into a final whole-class discussion. Inevitably during this discussion someone asks, 'What happened to the girl?'

The film ends with a question to the audience directed towards their sense of responsibility to the issues raised. The fate of the girl is left unclear. This was a deliberate editorial decision, for too often self-harming remains an ongoing feature in a young person's 'real life' story.

The teacher and I reviewed the session as we cleared desks and prepared for the next lesson.

Employing dramatic distancing within the debate certainly supported greater participation amongst the class, and passionate and engaged responses to a delicate and sensitive subject. The teacher's knowledge of the lives of young people in her class surprised her, and me. I made a note to talk to the learning support assistant who left with the class, to ask for her views.

Later in the day, two of the young people from the class met me in the restaurant, and asked 'Can you make a film of what you can do to help self-harmers? We have some ideas.' 'One day', I offered, 'let's meet up and talk it over.'

There followed a brief discussion before they left for PE and I went to meet my next client. It felt like, together, we had shifted some of the 'guilt and secrecy' surrounding the subject of self-harming that day.

Bibliography

Best, R. (2006) 'Deliberate self-harm in adolescence: a challenge for schools', *British Journal of Guidance & Counselling*, 34 (2), 161–175.

Boal, A. (1992) *Games for Actors and Non-Actors*. London: Routledge.

Boal, A. (1993) *Theatre of the Oppressed.* New York: Theatre Communications Group.

Foucault, M. (1995) *Discipline and Punishment: the Birth of the Prison.* A. Sheridan, (Translator). New York: Vintage Books.

Hall, B., Elliott, J. and Place, M. (2010) 'Self-harm through cutting: evidence from a sample of schools in the north of England', *Pastoral Care in Education*, 28(1), 33–43.

Hanworth, K., Rodham, K. and Evans, E. (2002) *Youth and Self Harm: Perspectives – a report.* Centre for Suicide Research, University of Oxford. Available at: http://www.samaritans.org/pdf/Samaritans-YouthSelfHarmPerspectives-full.pdf (Accessed 4 January 2011).

Hawton, K., Fagg, J., Simkin, S., Bale, E. and Bond, A. (2000) 'Deliberate self-harm in adolescents in Oxford, 1985–1995', *Journal of Adolescence*, 23, 47–55.

Howes, D. (2003) *Sensual Relations: Engaging the Senses in Culture and Social Theory.* Ann Arbor: University of Michigan Press.

Jackson, T. (1993) *Learning Through Theatre: New Perspectives on Theatre in Education.* Routledge: London.

Kidger, J., Donavan, J., Biddle, L., Cambell, R. and Gunnel, D. (2009) *Supporting Adolescent Emotional Health in Schools: A Mixed Methods Study of Students and Staff Views in England.* BMC Public Health.

Klonsky, E. D. and Muehlenkamp, J. J. (2007) 'Self-injury: A research review for the practitioner', *Journal of Clinical Psychology*, 63, 1045–1056.

Lippard, L. (1997) *The Lure of the Local: Senses of Place in a Multicentered Society.* New York: The New Press.

McAllister, M. (2003) 'Multiple meanings of self harm: A critical review', *International Journal of Mental Health Nursing*, 12, 177–185.

Naylor, P. B., Cowie, H. A., Walters, S. J., Talamelli, L. and Dawkins, J. (2009) 'Impact of a mental health teaching programme on adolescents', *The British Journal of Psychiatry*, 194 (4), 365–370.

Social Care Institute for Excellence (2005) *Deliberate self-harm (DSH) among children and adolescents: who is at risk and how is it recognised?* SCIE research briefing 16. Available at: http://www.scie.org.uk/publications/briefings/briefing16/index.asp (Accessed 4 January 2011).

Shotter, J. and Katz, A. (1996) 'Articulating a practice from within the practice itself: Establishing formative dialogues by the use of a "social poetics"', *Concepts and Transformation*, 1(2–3), 213–237.

Winnicott, D. W. (1990) *Maturational Processes and the Facilitating Environment: Studies in the Theory of Emotional Development.* London: Karnac Books.

17 Play and reality in child psychosis: how psychoanalytical dramatherapy can open the door to the world of make believe

Tamar Brown

Introduction

This chapter will discuss the possible effects of therapeutic work with children, with particular attention to the influence it can have on their capacity to adjust to a school system. It is important to describe the cultural contexts within which the clinical work takes place, the understanding and recognition of dramatherapy and the particularities and differences of the education systems in France and in Great Britain. I will briefly discuss different approaches in the work with autistic and psychotic children and then focus on the area of play and reality, illustrated by clinical vignettes.

Play in dramatherapy can facilitate a clearer distinction between the imaginary world and reality. In cases of child psychosis, these two areas often seem blurred and indistinct (Bion 1967: 43–64). In a child's 'normal' development, play is a process by which children integrate a distinction between their inner world and their external environment. In varying forms of child psychosis the capacity to play can be hindered. Thoughts and actions are interpreted in a very literal way. Access to symbolic representation is not internalized. This can be illustrated by a lack of sense of humour for example, a tendency to extreme sensitivity and a feeling of being permeable to other people's perceptions and remarks. In psychosis, there is no substantial filter in place to protect oneself from outer stimulations and projections, which are easily experienced as attacking or persecutory.

Dramatherapy and psychoanalysis

I arrived in France as a trained dramatherapist in 1993 with the idea that a network of alternative therapies was in place and that there would be an interest in the use of dramatherapy. However, the approach to clinical work can be described as predominantly Cartesian, with an emphasis on an initial university training in clinical psychology, before it is possible to specialize in any other technique or approach. Once qualified as a clinical psychologist in the French system, I was hired as such and once in post I set up several dramatherapy groups. Dramatherapy is not generally recognized or practised in France, but there are several forms of clinical work using theatre as a therapeutic medium. Psychodrama practice is widely recognized.

In dramatherapy, each country's history of theatre and psychiatry equally influence its practice. Each dramatherapist identifies how he or she approaches the work: the method, the theoretical references, the techniques used, and the analysis of the clinical material. A model based on a combined approach of dramatherapy and psychoanalysis can enrich this scope to analyse and transform the material produced, in particular with the attention given to primary unconscious processes.

In France, psychoanalysis remains a significant influence in the field of psychiatry. Theories on groupwork and group dynamics developed by Didier Anzieu (1975), René Kaës (1993) and others are an important source in order to help think through the complex labyrinth of unconscious processes inherent in all groups. Anzieu (1975) talks specifically of the idea of 'enveloppes' of the skin, of sound, of the body, and the idea of a container that comes to hold or to envelop, allowing one's more archaic emotional experiences to develop into thoughts and thinking. In a group, there are 'enveloppes' that can be created not only on an individual level, but also on a group level. When working with children with psychotic characteristics or who are on the autistic spectrum, a tendency can be observed of a need to create an 'enveloppe' that occupies all of the mind space. This allows the maintaining of a certain sensation and blotting out relating to others. One example could be when a sound or a movement is recreated in a repetitive, constant manner, making all other forms of communication or contact very difficult. In this way there is the idea that the patient uses this form of 'enveloppe' predominantly as a defence mechanism against emotional pain.

Kaës (1993) refers to the concept of an 'internal group' that suggests that we have all integrated or introjected an internal group that then becomes a main source of influence and represents a part of our 'self'. In a dramatherapy group aspects of one's internal group can take form through what the group creates onstage. This reflects what can resonate on an unconscious level between one person's internal world and another's, and within the group. On a spontaneous level, what does the group choose to play? What are the common themes and the recurrent preoccupations, and how can these inform us about what the group is experiencing and where they are situated in terms of the group process? A psychoanalytic approach to dramatherapy in groups offers another reading of the group dynamics through the medium of play, taking into account in particular archaic processes that refer to primary, sensorial, not yet elaborated affects, inherent in all groups, these reflect those experienced in infancy as described by Klein (1988), Bion (1967),Tustin (1981) and Winnicott (1965, 1971). These can be defined as follows.

There are three fundamental forms of archaic anxieties present from the period of birth in 'normal' development and they are experienced as very powerful sensations: a sense of splitting into fragments, a sensation of falling, and a sensation of melting/breaking down. These are sensations linked to primary experiences at the time of birth and in particular during the first six months to a year of life. They are emotional states that are felt without yet being able to be thought about. They invade and overwhelm and represent disintegrated states of mind. In this first phase of life, Klein in *Notes on some schizoid mechanisms* (1946), describes this state as the paranoid-schizoid position. It is a state of fragmentation and persecution. The position that follows is described as the depressive position. It is thought that this process, enabling disparate thoughts and feelings to be linked between each other, is made possible through a 'good enough' relationship and capacity for attunement between the infant and his or her environment. When this transition between an internal sense of fragmentation and a more integrated state of mind has not been sufficiently elaborated, it can contribute to cases of pathologies linked to psychosis. This signifies that it has not been possible to access and tolerate sufficiently the depressive position. Therefore, these archaic anxieties continue to be experienced throughout life, in particular at moments of great distress. Bion (1967) further developed Klein's (1946) theory when describing ego splitting, a process that prevents the self from being experienced as unified. Instead it is experienced as something that can be split into fragments. Hannah Segal comments that 'the containment of anxiety is the beginning of mental stability and also the basic model for the therapeutic endeavour of the analyst' (cited in Sinason 1992: 81). It is interesting to make a link between these theories and the dramatherapy concept of role repertoire. In the cases of psychosis and autism, one could say that the role repertoire and the capacity to adapt one's role to a particular situation is more restricted. This will be explained further as the chapter develops.

It is similar to the tendency to freeze one's emotional states or to limit one's environment in order to avoid over-stimulation. In this context, dramatherapy becomes a very useful technique for developing and extending one's role repertoire through exploring and experimenting with unfamiliar roles in the safety of the play space.

Different approaches to clinical work with children on the autism spectrum and children with psychotic characteristics

Autism and psychosis have often been at the heart of great controversy in terms of their origins, the causes and the varying approaches to treatment. In autism, there is a severe withdrawal from reality, with very little awareness of others. In psychosis, the imaginary world is very present, but there is considerably more interaction with the external world. There is less of a sense of an encapsulated world in which there is no or very little access, as in autism. At a conference in Avignon, France, in 2009, entitled '8ièmes rencontre entre le corps et psyche, Congès International "L'enfant autiste et on corps"') ('Eighth meeting between body and mind, International congress "The autistic child and his/her body"'), it was very reassuring to find that bridges were being built between psychoanalysis, neurosciences and educational models. There seems to be a realization that, due to the complexity of the pathologies, they need a number of different but complementary interventions are needed, and that one unique form of treatment does not exist. Research in the field of the neurosciences suggests that in autism it is very complicated to sustain several forms of stimulation simultaneously. Consequently, patients can spend a great deal of energy and time maintaining only one kind of sensation. This hypothesis is very helpful in helping to make sense of qualities of behaviour that can appear 'stuck' and restricted. In her book *Live Company*, child psychotherapist Alvarez (1992) stresses the importance of being able to resist the tendency in autism to deaden thought, by the therapist staying very much alive and continuing to think and offer openings for patients in order to accompany them to gradually 'unfreeze' their capacity for thinking. She describes this as an awakening process, and likens it to a glacier melting. Like a glacier, 'this may bring in its train huge cascades of emotion which the child may find difficult to regulate; in other forms of autism, the "deep freeze" as one patient of mine called it, may be much slower to thaw' (1992: 62).

Freezing emotional states to avoid feeling what can be experienced as unbearable emotional pain can take the form of withdrawal or manic activity, which can be witnessed in autism and psychosis. Alvarez underlines 'the distinction between the manic defence and the "manic position", that is, between states of mind which signal denial of unhappiness and those which signal escape from or emergence from such states into something like happiness' (1999: 127).

Play and reality, and the role of dramatherapy

Winnicott stated that we should think about the preoccupations of the young child playing: 'What matters is the near-withdrawal state . . . This area of playing is not inner psychic reality. It is outside the individual, but it is not the external world' (1971: 51).

It is this very particular state between two worlds in which, on the one hand, the child is able to develop his or her self, and his or her capacity to think, and on the other, it is a state which he or she does not control, where, through suspended belief, inner thoughts can be transformed. Robert Landy states, 'Although a wide range of play theories has developed, a certain commonality exists. The common denominator is the dramatic nature of play in the sense of drama as a dialectic between the actual, everyday reality and the imaginative one' (1986: 63). It is in this in-between terrain (similar to Winnicott's (1971) description of the transitional space), that new options, new roles can be explored in 'make believe' without the risk of consequences to everyday reality.

I would like to illustrate this with a clinical example that involves a psychoanalytical approach to dramatherapy.

A dramatherapy group in France

In a day hospital in Southern France, children between the ages of 2 and 12 are integrated into mainstream or specialized schooling, and, on a part-time basis, they are referred for treatment. A law established in 2005 was implemented in France making it compulsory for the education system to integrate all children with special needs. These children have assistance in the form of an 'aide à la vie sociale': a worker to help them on an individual basis to follow the classes, to accompany them to participate in various aspects of everyday social life. There are regular meetings between the educational staff, health workers and parents in order to exchange on the progress, the difficulties of the child, and to adjust the project according to these exchanges. At times staff from the hospital make observations in class, accompanying the child to and from school, or they meet up individually with a teacher who may be experiencing difficulties in understanding and managing a child's behaviour. Health workers such as psychiatric nurses, 'éducateurs' (a profession that does not exist in the UK, which works on the boundary between adapting social behaviour and taking into consideration emotional needs and the effects of different pathologies), can offer some insight and guidelines if necessary. All children are referred through the local child and family centre. The day hospital is multidisciplinary with psychiatric nurses, educators, speech therapist, psychomotricienne (a profession that does not exist in the UK, which highlights the link between body and mind), social worker, clinical psychologist, child psychiatrist, secretary and housekeeper.

The children come to the day hospital between one and five half-days a week. They each have a key worker and following an observation period, an individual project is established detailing which groups they will participate in and whether they will also be offered individual therapy or speech therapy or work focusing on body movement and awareness. As a clinical psychologist I did clinical evaluations of each child, I offered individual child therapy and I worked with the parents of these children, and helped team members to reflect on the groups they ran. I also participated in team meetings with the aim of contributing a clinical perspective on case studies and specific projects.

A dramatherapy group was set up in addition to a wide variety of groups already in place, with an emphasis on role play and improvization for a small group of children who displayed psychotic characteristics in their behaviour. The group demonstrated their inability to filter stimulation and their tendency to be highly influenced by each other's behaviour. There was a great deal of imitation and an adhesive manner of relating. An adhesive identification (Esther Bick, 1968) is linked to the experience of early interactions between infant and mother when 'a two-dimensional sticking-of-the-self-onto-the-other develops' (Waddell 1998: 107), and is maintained as a way of relating to others. It was also noted that there was a fluctuation in the children's behaviour from 'manic' states to more withdrawn states. The initial phase of this group was dominated by what could be described as this 'manic' state offstage. It was as though the children had to be in a permanent state of movement, to the point of getting into a sort of 'frenzy'; that they gave the impression of losing a sense of their body boundaries in a search to collide, to push the limits of what was acceptable physical contact with each other. This 'manic' state was coupled with moments where the children would withdraw. They expressed an absence of ideas when asked to invent a scene or they would get into a foetal position, stop the constant movement, and seem to seek comfort in the form of physical contact with the therapists. At times the children also seemed beyond reach, caught up in their 'frenzy', their closed inner world. When invited to create a scenario onstage, the children wanted to play magical dinosaurs, birds, robots, omnipotent creatures that could destroy anything potentially threatening. However, although able to imagine themselves as a creature, for instance, co-creating a scene together was notably impossible because each creature wanted to dominate and direct the other roles.

Scenarios and the use of a fairy tale (which includes themes around abandonment, individuation, survival) were suggested by the therapists, who could also participate in the scenes. During the second term, with this input, themes such as fraternal rivalry, abandonment, death, infantile fears such as murderous desires, helplessness and dependency were prevalent. There was still a desire in the children to play imaginary creatures. There was also now a new possibility of playing reality-based stories. The initial state of 'frenzy' of the group seemed to evoke on the one hand that the group could be experienced as dangerous, and on the other that thoughts that might come to mind had to be fervently chased away, by keeping the body active.

Less defensive, more hopeful states

Although the children showed a certain resistance to the therapists suggesting the content of the scenes, having that context seemed to act as a filter that adjusted the levels of excitement, whilst at the same time permitting them to explore issues that seemed to preoccupy them as children. It was as though the 'manic' state offstage could be transformed into a more 'manic position' onstage (Klein 1935), in other words, it could be less in the form of a defence and more in a newly discovered sense of hope (Alvarez 1992). During some of the scenes it seemed possible momentarily for the children to stay with depressive feelings, when, for example, it was imagined in a scenario that a baby was suddenly left alone; or a fear could be acknowledged that parents could contemplate abandoning their children in the forest.

In the third term and beginning of the second year, the capacity in these children to bear depressive feelings onstage and to feel held in the mind of the therapists seemed to allow a shift into a more expansive role repertoire. For example, Henry, eight years old, at the beginning of this work could only play objects and particularly 'unlikeable' objects that invited rejection, such as a bit of snot or a part of an animal. He was indecisive and seemed to be void of ideas. Through the psychodramatic technique of the 'voice-off', he was able to lean on the thinking capacity of the therapist and the group to develop his own thinking processes. This process of transforming a feeling/sensation into a bearable thought has a parallel with Bion's description of the alpha function (Bion 1962). Henry suddenly seemed to inhabit, to play the role in interaction with the other roles. It gave the impression that he was able to let go of himself for that short moment in order to try and imagine himself as somebody else, and in so doing paradoxically become a little bit more his authentic self. From then on, he was able to humanize the parts he played and to differentiate a little bit more between play and reality.

Conclusion

Within the school framework, teachers and schools were often challenged by the 'manic' states in which the children from the group could get held up. One could hypothesize that over a longer span of time, this kind of work could facilitate and contribute to preventive work. A dramatherapy group in the context described appears to help children to internalize a more stable container to moderate greater levels of anxiety.

To conclude, there remains a certain enigma as to what happens on stage that allows the child a different way of being. The stage seems to act as a container of emotions just under the surface, allowing an adaptation to the invented situation and an ability to create. The fact that onstage therapist and patients also share a play space invites the possibility of entering the imaginary world of the patients, without it being intrusive, as Winnicott (1971) underlined. This encourages the establishment of a certain intimacy, and it remains safe because of the 'enveloppe' provided by the group. The freedom of anything being possible to play onstage is also an important factor. Within this freedom of make-believe, it seems that children with psychotic characteristics can take the risk of being more in touch with realistic scenarios. Being offered these opportunities within school seems an effective way of filtering overwhelming feelings, containing them and therefore allowing the children to be more accessible for future learning within school's more structured, restrictive boundaries. In this group it seemed that playing and make-believe within an on stage environment created a higher tolerance for experiencing and staying with certain depressive feelings.

Play in child development is the means by which one differentiates reality and make-believe, self and other, inner and outer worlds. In psychosis this is not clearly established and the boundaries often remain blurred and often confused. Offering the opportunity to revisit this process through dramatherapy can encourage bringing back to life parts of the self, roles that have not been sufficiently inhabited, and allow the assembling of fragmented split parts.

Preventive work in schools can help to restore these capacities and prevent more severe pathologies taking root. Offering a safe, playful space for children to explore troubled aspects of their internal world can be extremely beneficial. It can create new openings to avoid inner conflicts becoming permanent or chronic features. School is representative of a 'normal', 'healthy' environment that promotes knowledge and growth. It is a much more accessible and neutral setting than a specific mental health centre, which can carry many taboos and negative connotations for the larger public. School can be seen as an intermediary space in which the child maintains his or her place and a sense of belonging, whilst in a sort of 'annexe zone' they can explore areas of emotional difficulty.

In *Inside Lives*, child psychotherapist Waddell (1998) describes the growth of the personality and she quotes Bion: 'Learning depends on the capacity for (the growing container) to remain integrated and yet lose rigidity. This is the foundation of the state of mind of the individual who can retain his knowledge and experience and yet be prepared to reconstrue past experiences in a manner that enables him to be receptive of a new idea' (Bion in Waddell 1998: 103).

This quote illustrates the extent to which dramatherapy and psychoanalysis link up with each other. It stresses the necessity for a certain elasticity within thinking, necessary for the growth of the personality to take place.

Bibliography

Alvarez, A. (1992) *Live Company*. London: Routledge.
Anzieu, D. (1975) *Le groupe et l'inconscient*. Paris: Dunod.
Anzieu, D. (1985) *Le Moi Peau*. Paris: Dunod.
Avron, O. (1996) *La Pensée Scénique*. Ramonville, Saint-Agne: Editions Erès.
Bick, E. (1968) 'The experience of the skin in early object-relations', *International Journal of Psycho-Analysis* 49, 484–486.
Bion, W.R. (1962) 'The psycho-analytic study of thinking', *International Journal of Psycho-Analysis* 43, 306–310.
Bion, W. (1967) *Second Thoughts*. London, William Heinemann Medical Books.
Casement, P. (1985) *On Learning from the Patient*. London: Tavistock.
Houzel, D. (2001) 'The "nest of babies" fantasy', *Journal of Child Psychotherapy* 27 (2), 125–138.
Jones, P. (2007) *Drama as Therapy* (second edition). East Sussex: Routledge.
Kaës, R. (1993) *Le Groupe et le sujet du groupe*. Paris: Dunod.
Klein, M. (1935) 'A contribution to the psychogenesis of manic depressive states', *International Journal of Psycho-Analysis* 16, 145–174.

Klein, M. (1946) 'Notes on some schizoid mechanisms', *International Journal of Psycho-Analysis* xxvii, 99–110.
Klein, M. (1988) *Love, Guilt and Reparation*. London: Virago Press.
Landy, R. J. (1986) *Drama Therapy*. Springfield IL: Charles C. Thomas.
Maher, M. (1975) *The Psychological Birth of the Human Infant: Symbiosis and Individuation*. Great Britain: Hutchinson and Co.
Segal, H. (1964) *Introduction to the Work of Melanie Klein*. London: The Hogarth Press Ltd.
Sinason, V. (1992) *Mental Handicap and the Human Condition, New Approaches from the Tavistock*. London: Free Association Books.
Tustin, F. (1981) *Autistic States in Children*. London: Routledge.
Waddell, M. (1998) *Inside Lives*. London: Tavistock Clinic Series.
Winnicott, D.W. (1965) *The Maturational Processes and the Facilitating Environment*. London: The Hogarth Press.
Winnicott, D.W. (1971) *Playing and Reality*. London: Pelican.

18 The charity Roundabout: one model of providing dramatherapy in schools

Deborah Haythorne

Introduction

This chapter looks at the charity Roundabout and how it provides dramatherapy in schools. It briefly traces the history of the organization and its growth with regard to schools provision. It refers to how Roundabout sets up new provision within schools and describes the different groups of children and young people that Roundabout works with. The chapter includes quotes from service users, parents, carers and teachers, all of whom have given consent for publication.

Roundabout – the beginning

Lynn Cedar and Deborah Haythorne (the author) founded Roundabout in 1985. It became a registered charity in 1987 (charity no. 297491), with a remit to provide educational, psychological and artistic benefit to a wide range of disadvantaged people throughout London, through the provision of a dramatherapy service. At this time, there was very little dramatherapy provision in the UK and virtually no established posts for which dramatherapists could apply. Setting up a 'not for profit' organization in the voluntary sector was a proactive and creative response to this challenge, but it also meant taking a step into the unknown for the founders and indeed the profession. Roundabout had few role models to draw on and the founders began a steep learning curve.

The aim of the charity was to discover unmet needs that dramatherapy could potentially address within the community. Roundabout's initial service users included adults with learning disabilities, adults with acute and chronic mental health needs and children with autistic spectrum disorder. The charity grew as a result of advertising and word of mouth. Growth depended on funding and although Roundabout made a charge for its services, many potential service user groups were financially disadvantaged. Roundabout sought both core funding in order to support the development of the charity and project funding to cover its work with different service user groups in the various settings. A core grant from the Association of

London Governments (now known as the London Councils) in 1987 created opportunities for Roundabout to expand and employ more drama-therapists. Further project grants followed and Roundabout began to widen its range of service user groups and increase the number of boroughs in which it was able to offer its services. A grant from the Big Lottery Fund in 1999 enabled Roundabout to set up a second office base in Islington, in addition to the main office in Croydon. This led to a large increase in provision, particularly over the following six years.

This careful, slow, steady development has led to Roundabout becoming the UK's leading voluntary sector dramatherapy service provider. The two founders have remained with the charity throughout, becoming the project directors, and many of the current staff have worked with Roundabout over a number of years. Roundabout staff have contributed greatly to the development of dramatherapy in the UK and taken on a number of significant roles from training students to representing the dramatherapy profession at international conferences.

Roundabout – growth

In 2010 Roundabout celebrated its Silver Jubilee, recognizing 25 years of dramatherapy service provision. The charity has continued to grow and the 2009/2010 Roundabout Annual Report made reference to work in 13 London Boroughs and two local authorities outside London. There were 52 different weekly projects during the year and Roundabout worked with 49 different organizations, including 39 schools, five residential homes, two day centres and three support groups. It worked with 21 different service user groups, 684 service users between the ages of 3 and over 90, and 40 per cent of those service users were from black and minority ethnic backgrounds. Roundabout's team of employed and freelance dramatherapists facilitated the projects, supported by the project directors, the administration team and the charity's trustees.

Roundabout – schools

Since the charity started, the project directors have always prioritized work with children in schools. Initially much of the school-based work was a result of parents and carers contacting Roundabout directly after finding information about the charity in a directory of services, or from a personal contact, or more recently on our website. Their enquiry was usually about how dramatherapy could benefit their child and this occasionally resulted in individual sessions, usually in a child's own home. However, more often, it resulted in Roundabout setting up a new project in the child's school.

There are a number of reasons why the school may provide the best context for the work. Very often, when a parent is explaining why they are interested in dramatherapy for their child, the child's issues have a social/

peer factor that would be best addressed within a group setting or within the environment where those factors are present. This can be of particular relevance to children with autistic spectrum disorder because 'interactions that require the children to focus on peers create a positive social group culture. Within this culture and environment, self-awareness and positive self-esteem can be fostered' (Krasny et al. 2003: 107).

The child may be experiencing difficulties within the school environment and accessing dramatherapy in school can support the child's whole experience of school. These factors are explored further in a number of other chapters in this book. Children can be tired at the end of the school day and dramatherapy provision after school or at the weekend can intrude on family time. Scheduling sessions during the school day is generally better for the child's well-being. Teaching staff and parents or carers usually support children coming out of class to attend dramatherapy sessions if the time of the sessions is carefully and sensitively negotiated.

> Whilst the work involved the children being withdrawn from their classes, there is no doubt that every child derived huge benefits from receiving dramatherapy. My teachers fully supported the work of the team and acknowledged the positive impact it had, not just for the individual child but also the other children and staff involved. Noted benefits were in children's relationships with their peers and with adults.
>
> (Head teacher of a primary school)

Where referral issues for a child or young person focus on home and family life, again experience has shown that very often the school environment can provide a familiar safe place for these issues to be explored through the dramatherapy. The sessions can provide a focus of support for cooperative working between family, school and other professional services that may be involved in the child or young person's care provision. Inevitably, financial considerations are often another reason for recommending that a child or young person should access dramatherapy through their school. The cost of ongoing dramatherapy sessions on a private basis may be prohibitive for the family.

The most important step after the first contact is to arrange a face-to-face meeting with Roundabout staff visiting the school. This is important, regardless of the availability of potential funds for the project, because funding cannot be found until the need for and shape of the project has been established. At this first stage, it is important to establish whether Roundabout can offer something additional to the school, over and beyond what they already can and do provide. As Professor Irvine Gersch pointed out in his Keynote address at the British Association of Dramatherapists (BADth) annual conference 2001:

> children might be helped considerably through Dramatherapy, as an additional provision for selected students. Such provision could serve to enhance the school's assessment of special needs and it could provide information for teachers to use in their work with children, for example, ideas about behaviour management. . .
>
> (Gersch 2001: 6)

Roundabout – funding

Roundabout's main source of income is derived from fees and grants, with additional funding from statutory bodies like local authorities and donations. Funding for Roundabout's work in schools usually comes from a combination of grants and fees. A pilot project may be funded by a grant, which either allows the service to be offered for free or at a discounted price. Sessions may be offered for a half a day or a full day, with the school receiving sessions from one or maybe two dramatherapists. The dramatherapists offer sessions for groups and individuals and the projects are evaluated by the dramatherapists and the school at the end of the pilot. Many times pilot projects have developed into long-term relationships with the schools, where the school has taken on the cost of the sessions and made a commitment to a long-term relationship with Roundabout.

In 2006/2007 Roundabout worked in two nursery schools, six primary schools and five secondary schools. By 2009/2010 Roundabout was working in nine nursery schools, twenty primary schools and ten secondary schools. Roundabout was able to extend its work because of an increased demand and in particular through working with extended schools funding. This funding allowed Roundabout to work with three different clusters of schools brought together by their geographical proximity. These school clusters of between six and twelve schools each independently recognized the need for therapeutic services within their schools and worked together to jointly commission therapy services that could be shared between the schools within the clusters. One Roundabout dramatherapist might therefore find themselves working in four different local schools over a period of three days, including time to meet with their supervisor at the Roundabout office.

Roundabout – a case study

Roundabout received a phone call from a parent who thought that dramatherapy might benefit her primary school-aged child with autistic spectrum disorder (ASD). During the first telephone conversation with the mother, the Roundabout Project Director proposed sending her information about Roundabout, i.e. annual report and the fee sheet, and she agreed to approach the Special Educational Needs Coordinator (SENCO) at her child's school, armed with the information about Roundabout and dramatherapy, to see if they would be interested in Roundabout working in the school. The SENCO was interested and Roundabout and the mother arranged to visit the school. When a project starts in this way, the relationship with the school is based on a shared concern for the child in question.

When one of Roundabout's project directors attended the meeting, she found that the SENCO had already begun to identify other children who might benefit from dramatherapy, based on the information the mother had given them. The SENCO and the child's mother felt that because the child was experiencing difficulties developing positive peer relationships and had poor confidence and self-esteem, it would be helpful to first offer them one-to-one sessions with the longer term aim of offering dramatherapy sessions with a small group of peers. After consultation with the head teacher and bursar, the SENCO proposed that the school should receive a six-week pilot project for half a day each week, with the initial child receiving one-to-one sessions with the dramatherapist who would also work with two groups of children from the school, including children with ASD, learning difficulties and other referral reasons.

The project was well received and the children were all seen to benefit from the dramatherapy sessions. The school extended the project and ended up committing to two years of dramatherapy. The SENCO told other schools in the same borough about the project and Roundabout ended up working in four other primary schools in the same borough. All this from one phone call from a concerned mother.

> The dramatherapists, by their calm approach and enthusiasm to encourage self expression, have brought much joy to him and brought on his confidence and relationships with his peers.
>
> (Parent of primary school child)

Roundabout – ongoing work

Once a project in a school is established, the key to continuing success is good communication with the children and young people, the school staff and the parents and carers. Roundabout dedicates time to discussing the potential of the project in the school, the way in which it might fit in with the school's ethos and timetable, the importance of identifying appropriate adults for the dramatherapists to liaise with, and most importantly, identifying the individual children who might benefit.

> Their insight and concern for the children matches our priority for social and emotional development, and they also have a very realistic and practical approach to expectations. Their feed-back is invaluable.
>
> (Teacher in secondary school)

In Roundabout's early days there was a tendency to rush into a project, trying to ensure that the dramatherapy was offered to as many children as possible. The team were concerned to spread accessibility as widely as possible, and wanted to show that the service offered value for money. Since then Roundabout has learnt that by taking more time to carefully explain the nature of dramatherapy, the referrer is able to make considered and appropriate choices for group and individual dramatherapy sessions. Spreading the service too thinly decreases the potential impact. Although the result may well be the creation of a waiting list for dramatherapy, this should not be seen as something negative.

> Any child who is experiencing distress for whatever reason cannot realistically be expected to benefit fully from the curriculum on offer unless we can help such distress to be alleviated. I believe that Roundabout dramatherapists achieved this. The dramatherapy enabled each child to find the space to confront their trauma and the experienced support of the therapists ensured they were able to work towards dealing with this very stressful time in their lives.
>
> (Inclusion officer at a primary school)

It would be impossible to overstate the importance of well-planned, regular liaison with a named member of staff. Roundabout always proposes that this take place before and after the sessions each week. It is also very important, at the start of a project, to identify suitable documentation relating to a new project. To ensure this happens, Roundabout uses a project start-up pack, which covers the development of a service agreement, the British Association of Dramatherapists (BADth) Code of Ethical Practice, and various policies, such as Roundabout's Safeguarding Policy for Children and Young People and the Roundabout policy on working with touch.

Parents are asked by the school to consent to their child attending dramatherapy. Roundabout always proposes that the dramatherapists start by observing referred children in class, assessing them individually, and meeting class teachers and parents. Last, but by no means least, the children are always asked directly, in an accessible and appropriate way, whether or not they would like to attend dramatherapy.

Roundabout – who benefits from dramatherapy?

Whilst it is fair to comment that more detailed research is required, our experience has shown us, time after time, that the medium of dramatherapy is particularly effective with children and young people because of its appeal, immediacy and accessibility. In Roundabout's experience, children often find it hard to express themselves through words; as a result, talking therapies and counselling may not suit everyone. Because dramatherapy works obliquely, using art forms such as stories and role-play, and uses non-verbal, as well as verbal means of communication, it can overcome this potential difficulty. As Watts writes, 'The expression of feeling in role can be a safe and creative way of acknowledging feelings so that we can learn to contain and finally have some choice in the way we express them' (1996: 33).

Dramatherapists have recorded in their reports, and observed, that using the language of metaphor and symbol, and using drama techniques such as story telling and role-play, children and young people can effectively express their thoughts and feelings, and their needs and issues. Cattanach, in her discussion of dramatic play with children, states:

> The Dramatherapist working with children uses dramatic play to help them make transformations of their experiences which enable them to make a shift in their experience. This is the core of drama as a healing process and is experienced when we move from everyday reality into dramatic reality.
>
> (1994: 138)

The dramatherapy sessions are accessible to many different children and young people. This includes those who might struggle to engage with school-based child support networks or counselling or talking therapies. With its non-direct and non-confrontational gentle approach, children and young people with learning difficulties, ASD, hearing and visual impairments, attention deficit hyperactivity disorder as well as children with low self-esteem, high anxiety and those who have experienced abuse have benefited from Roundabout's dramatherapy services. Dramatherapy as a profession would benefit from further evaluative studies to create a more extensive evidence base to support these claims.

> The world is a complex place for my son; to access a creative environment run by people skilled enough to understand him is wonderful.
>
> (Parent of child with ASD)

Roundabout also works with children and young people who have been identified as having low-level mental health needs because of their experience of issues such as neglect, alcoholism, bullying, family breakdown, bereavement, transition to a different school and change. Some of the children and young people are on the child protection register or are identified as a child in need and may come from dysfunctional family situations. Often they are struggling both academically and socially within the school.

> They [the dramatherapists] bring a new dimension to understanding children and how feelings and emotions affect learning. The therapy has linked very well with our work on the SEAL curriculum and is a

> fantastic forum for the children involved to release themselves in a safe and secure environment which the classroom can never provide.
>
> (Teacher in a primary school)

Over the years we have seen a wide variety of children each benefiting in their own unique way from their dramatherapy sessions. Sometimes the dramatherapists are lucky enough to hear them express this in their own words.

> My favourite lesson is dramatherapy because I like to make up my own stories. I like running around the hall and sometimes I use my imagination and pretend there's stuff like cars, swimming pools, food and even big television and I pretend that I'm wearing different clothes like wrestling attire, masks, hats and I pretend I'm other people . . . But we do have to take our shoes off when we go in to the hall but we don't have to take our socks off . . . Sometimes the dramatherapist asks me how my weekend was and I like to get the story started, but it takes a while, but in the end he gets me to say my news, then he will try and say his news, but I keep saying to him let's just get the story started. I love the stories because I get to tell them and act in them. At the end we will say what's your favourite bit.
>
> (15-year-old boy with Asperger's syndrome)

Observations of the benefits of dramatherapy are recorded in the dramatherapist's notes and reports, and through feed-back from SENCOs and teachers.

> There was also an improvement in the children's attendance and in their ability to access the curriculum and hence increased attainment. Changes were also noted in their self-esteem and with it their ability to acknowledge their own achievements and build on them.
>
> (SENCO from primary school)

Roundabout also implements a number of user evaluation systems, for example 'PSYCHLOPS Kids' described in chapter 19.

Roundabout – the future of work in schools

This chapter has presented one model of dramatherapy provision in schools. Meldrum (chapter 23) sets out another model and some specific guidelines for setting up dramatherapy projects in schools.

Roundabout provides services that are being received enthusiastically by the children and young people it serves and by the schools it works in partnership with. This successful model has been an inspiration to other dramatherapists and one role for Roundabout in the future may be to develop satellite projects elsewhere in the UK.

Working as a voluntary sector organization within the community, Roundabout is very strongly placed to lead the way for the art therapies to raise their profile with regard to the Government's 'Big Society' plan. David Cameron (2010) stated that Big Society is about 'social action', 'public service reform' and 'community empowerment' through 'decentralisation', 'transparency' and 'finance'. As the local community takes on more responsibility and power to determine local services to local people, dramatherapists need to speak out about the services they can offer.

Also relevant to this thinking is that the schools White Paper *The Importance of Teaching* (Department for Education 2010) sets out a radical reform programme for the schools system, with schools apparently freed from the constraints of central government direction, and placing teachers firmly at the heart of school improvement. Dramatherapists already work closely with teachers to help improve children and young people's lives and learning experiences. It may be that some schools will choose to spend their Pupil Premium to bring in dramatherapy services to support pupils with additional needs related to social deprivation.

Whatever happens in local and national government, it is clear that dramatherapy has a place in schools and dramatherapists have a role to play in helping to improve the lives of children and young people. Roundabout will continue to strive to support this process through providing their services to those who need them most.

> The provision of drama therapy by Roundabout has been extremely important as it has added another dimension to the pupils' learning that is sadly not available through the national curriculum. The benefits of drama therapy for the children have been invaluable, by removing them from the curriculum for one lesson they are more able to access the curriculum for the remainder of the week . . . The pupils obviously enjoy their time with you and we see a marked improvement in their skills elsewhere in the school.
>
> (Head teacher secondary school)

References

Cameron, D. (2010) *Our Big Society Agenda*. Available at: http://www.conservatives.com/News/Speeches/2010/07/David_Cameron_Our_Big_Society_Agenda.aspx (accessed 31 December 2010).

Cattanach, A. (1994) 'Dramatic play with children – The interface of dramatherapy and play therapy', in Jennings, S., Cattanach, A., Mitchell, S., Chesner, A. and Meldrum, B. (eds.), *The Handbook of Dramatherapy*. London: Routledge.

Department for Education (2010) *The Importance of Teaching: Schools White Paper*.

Available at: http://www.education.gov.uk/schools/teachingandlearning/schoolswhitepaper/b0068570/the-importance-of-teaching (accessed 31 December 2010).

Gersch, I. S. (2001) 'Dramatherapy in education: opportunities for the future: a view from the outside', *Dramatherapy (Special 'Education' Edition)* 23(1), 4–8.

Krasny, L., Williams, B. J., Provencal, S. and Ozonoff, S. (2003) 'Social skills interventions for the autism spectrum: essential ingredients and a model curriculum', *Child and Adolescent Psychiatric Clinics of North America* 12(1), 107–122.

Watts, P. (1996) 'Working with myth and story', in Pearson, J. (ed.), *Discovering the Self through Drama and Movement – The Sesame Approach*. London: Jessica Kingsley.

Part IV

Evidence and outcomes

19 Roundabout and the development of PSYCHLOPS Kids evaluation

Deborah Haythorne, Susan Crockford and Emma Godfrey

> There are many routes to apprehending, describing and knowing oneself or another. For Dramatherapy, a part of the way the therapist tries to know others is through assessment. Another aspect of this process concerns the way in which we try to understand what has happened over a period of time within the Dramatherapy – this is evaluation.
>
> (Jones 2007: 285)

Introduction

Evaluation is key to developing a high-quality, user-focused, needs-driven dramatherapy service. Dramatherapists need to be implementing before and after measures in all of their work in order to formalize this process of evaluation, and to create qualitative and quantitative data that can serve to ensure services are meeting the needs of service users. Dramatherapists also need user evaluation and feedback in order to develop their own practice (Barham 1999). In the current climate, evidence-based practice (EBP) is central to securing funding for dramatherapy, now and in the future. For example, the National Institute for Health and Clinical Excellence (2008) recommends that only school-based interventions that have proven effective should be provided in primary schools to help children identified as having social and emotional problems. This chapter will describe the development and piloting of a new measure to assess the outcome of dramatherapy interventions in schools.

The charity Roundabout holds a unique position within the dramatherapy community, as it is the leading service provider in the voluntary sector and brings together the largest number of dramatherapists working as a team in the UK. Lynn Cedar and Deborah Haythorne founded Roundabout in 1985 and they currently work with a team of 20 dramatherapists, eight of whom are employed while the remainder work as freelance dramatherapists. Roundabout offers its services to a wide geographical area that includes the whole of Greater London as well as some boroughs just outside London. They work with people of all ages and with a range of needs. Roundabout usually provides dramatherapy on a weekly basis to groups and individuals for an agreed period of time that can vary from 6 weeks to a number of years. In 2009/2010 Roundabout ran 52 weekly projects with 21 different service user groups. Out of these projects, 42 of them were with children and young people, and of these 39 took place in schools.

Background

For a number of years Roundabout has explored ways of eliciting service user feedback as a way of evaluating its services. Due to the charity's broad user base, this means that a number of methods are needed in order to ensure there is an appropriate and accessible methodology for each client group (Grainger 1999).

During 2008–09 Roundabout undertook an audit of its user feedback methods across all of its work, which identified a lack of suitable methods, particularly for children and young people. Roundabout widened the search by consulting with the wider dramatherapy community to discover what methods were being used by other dramatherapists with this age group. The main method being used was the 'Strengths and Difficulties Questionnaire' (SDQ, Goodman et al. 1998). This method is for children and young people aged 3–17 years. It has parent and teacher questionnaires and the opportunity for self-completion by 11–17-year-olds. The other measure that is widely used in a mental health setting such as Child and Adolescent Mental Health Services (CAMHS) is the Health of the Nation Outcome Scales for Children and Adolescents (HoNOSCA, Gowers et al. 1999). This is mainly clinician-rated and assesses behaviours, impairments, symptoms, and social functioning. There is a short self-report version available for adolescents for use alongside the clinician ratings.

The self-report instruments available, therefore, were for young people over the age of 11 years, which suggested there was a need to develop a self-report measure for children. This especially interested Roundabout, as they had been developing their own self-reporting pre- and post-therapy evaluation document for primary-aged children, called 'Three Wishes'. As Karkou (2010) has noted, it is particularly important to give children a voice because often they are excluded from the feedback process. 'A high proportion of studies on children and adolescents do not include responses from the children themselves, relying instead on the perceptions of parents, teachers or therapists. . .' (Karkou 2010: 95).

The development of 'PSYCHLOPS Kids'

In order to develop this methodology, Roundabout recognized the need to seek expert help in the form of a collaborative study (Karkou 2010) and to fundraise for the resources to action such a study.

In 2007 Roundabout began working with dramatherapist and psychologist Dr Godfrey to develop a new self-report method for children taking part in dramatherapy. Alongside this collaboration Roundabout built relationships with funders to support this work, resulting in substantial grants from the Terpsichore Trust and The Wates Foundation.

Dr Godfrey was one of a group of researchers with an interest in primary care mental health, formed in 1999 as part of South Thames Primary Care Research Network, London (STaRNET). It consisted of clinical psychologists, counselling psychologists, psychotherapists, counsellors, general practitioners, and academic mental health researchers from King's College London. The aim of this group was to investigate client-generated outcome measures and encourage user involvement in research. This type of questionnaire measures factors that are defined by the client, who is seen as the expert in issues of importance to them, rather than factors selected by a group of researchers or professional experts. These measures are likely to be more sensitive to change than conventional, checklist-type questionnaires because they tap into issues of importance to the client, rather than merely offering a checklist of items, not all of which may be meaningful or relevant to the individual. The group devised a client-generated outcome measure called 'PSYCHLOPS' (Psychological Outcome Profiles, Ashworth et al. 2004), with user involvement from Depression Alliance, a UK charity for people affected by depression, providing information and support services. It was derived from MYMOP, which is a patient-generated outcome measure focusing primarily on physical health problems (Paterson 1996). The final version of the PSYCHLOPS questionnaire was awarded the Crystal Mark by the Plain English Campaign. Therapist feedback about using this new measure was very positive (Ashworth et al. 2005).

PSYCHLOPS is a brief, self-administered questionnaire designed for use in adult mental health (Ashworth et al. 2005). It is designed to capture the client's own perspective of their psychological distress. It asks them to describe and then score the problem that troubles them the most at the start of therapy. They score the problem on a six-point scale ranging from 'not at all affected' to 'severely affected'. Further questions ask for a description and scoring of any other problems, and to describe and score what they find hard to do as a result of their problems (a score of functioning). Following these three idiographic questions, the final question is a nomothetic question, asking the respondent to score their well-being using a six-point scale (Ashworth 2007). Idiographic measures investigate individuals in depth in order to gain a unique understanding of each individual's perspective by measuring a different item or domain for each participant. Nomothetic measures investigate large groups of people by measuring responses to standardized questions. This is in order to distinguish between individuals falling within the normal range of responses and those falling outside this range, who may then be classified as part of a clinical population of interest.

The follow-up questionnaire used at the end of therapy is similar. The researcher is required to transcribe the original responses to the three free-text questions into identical boxes on the follow-up questionnaire. The client then scores these same items again, using identical scales, and the well-being score is repeated.

Total scores are obtained by adding the individual six-point scores for the four questions, giving a maximum score of 20, with greater severity indicated by higher scores. The questionnaire has been tested for reliability and validated against two widely used measures, the Clinical Outcomes Routine Evaluation (CORE, Ashworth et al. 2007) and the Hospital Anxiety Depression Scale (HADS, Ashworth et al. 2009). It has been employed in a range of studies in primary care (Ashworth et al. 2007; Bakker et al. 2007; Schreuders et al. 2005; Verhoef et al. 2006) and is included as a recommended measure in the Outcomes Compendium of the National Institute for Mental Health in England, 2009 (it can be accessed through the website: www.psychlops.org.uk).

Roundabout and Dr Godfrey decided to adapt adult PSYCHLOPS, which is explained above, for children, as there was no appropriate self-complete measure available for the 7–13 age group. The aim was to stay true to adult PSYCHLOPS by including the child's perspective (qualitative) whilst measuring outcome (quantitative). Elements of creative assessment were included within a user-friendly measure of distress, suitable for children and young people.

An initial pilot was conducted with therapists and children working with Roundabout to enable the development of the 'Kids' version. This resulted in space for drawings and a colourful format, as well as the use of emoticon faces to help assess levels of distress. The text was also altered with the substitution of the word 'worried' for the word 'troubles', as children appeared to associate trouble with being 'in trouble'. Therefore the first question asked was 'What are you most worried about in your life at the moment? Please write in the box below and add drawings if you want to'. The other changes were the removal of the second problem question, which confused children, and the addition of questions to assess hopes and fears before therapy and a reflection on dramatherapy after therapy. The maximum score was therefore 12 (problem Qx1, function Qx1, well-being Qx1, each scored on a five-point scale), with greater severity indicated by higher scores.

It was clear that given the wide age range of the children taking part, some adult support was needed to complete PSYCHLOPS Kids, including importantly an explanation of confidentiality and assent to fill out the form (Jones and Ramsden 2011), parents having already given written consent for dramatherapy. The children completed the initial pilot study during the first and last dramatherapy session, with support from the dramatherapist. In the later pilot, a member of the school staff supported children in completing the form before the dramatherapy sessions started and after the last session. The reason for this change was to avoid any bias in responses (Payne 1993). The dramatherapists had by this time reported a number of difficulties with the form being completed during the sessions. The most frequently mentioned problem by the dramatherapists was the nature of the relationship between the child and the therapist. In the first session the child did not know the therapist and therefore this might have had an influence on what the child chose to reveal on their form, and at the end of the therapy the child might not want to offer anything other than positive comments, as the therapist was present.

Interestingly, school staff reported that there was also a benefit to them in supporting children while filling out the forms. For example, one wrote: 'As the person who identifies potential children for dramatherapy, I found it confirming to know that the child was anxious about the areas I had identified as being of concern'. Another wrote: 'The information was very useful as it gave an insight to some of the things that the children may be worrying about at home'.

After the last pilot, it became clear that it would be helpful to expand the information-gathering top sheet on the pre-therapy form to include clear instructions to the adult supporting the child filling out the form, for example 'Please sit with the child as they fill out the form and support them to answer the questions for themselves'.

Before the pilot studies, schools were asked to give consent for their staff and children to take part in the pilot project. Parents were written to and asked to complete a consent form and the children were asked verbally first if they would like to take part in dramatherapy and later if they would like to complete PSYCHLOPS Kids. During the pilot, all Roundabout dramatherapists working in mainstream schools with children aged 7–13 (school years 3–8) were trained to use PSYCHLOPS Kids and agreed to take part in the study. They consulted their schools about taking part in the process and verbally instructed the school staff in how to support a child completing a PSYCHLOPS Kids form. The dramatherapists were initially resistant to formally evaluating their work in such a structured way. This dilemma is reflected within the profession (Jones 2007). However, once they engaged with the process, contrary to expectations, they found that the information gained through the forms was a good way into the therapeutic work with the children.

> We were all concerned that an evaluation tool would feel intrusive or would seem unconnected with the dramatherapy itself, however it has proved in many cases to be an additional therapeutic tool and the children have generally seemed to be OK about completing the forms.
> (Dramatherapist)

Results

Children from 25 mainstream primary and secondary schools in Barnet, Croydon, Hammersmith and Fulham, Surbiton, Sutton and Westminster were enrolled in the pilot. Children were referred for various reasons. Most of these were for issues related to bullying, challenging behaviour or extreme shyness; some were for family difficulties. Fifty-eight pairs of pre- and post-questionnaires were completed and used as the basis for the results of this study. Of the 58 individuals who completed the forms, 23 were identified as white British, 14 were identified as coming from other ethnic groups and 21 did not have any ethnicity recorded on the form. Thirty-four (59 per cent) were boys and 24 (41 per cent) were girls. The average age of the sample was 10.2 years.

The average time between pre-therapy and follow-up assessment was 3 months. The average pre-therapy score at the start of dramatherapy was 5.7 (standard deviation [sd] 3.4), while the average post-therapy score was 3.1 (sd 2.7). Standard deviation is the measure of how much variance there is around the mean. This gave an effect size of 0.8 for the dramatherapy intervention. An effect size of 0.8 is generally considered to be large and indicates an effective intervention (Cohen 1988).

Two separate researchers independently undertook a thematic qualitative analysis of the first question about what children were most worried about. There were a number of themes identified. These were:

- School problems, including worries about tests, anxiety about school transfer, and general concerns about schoolwork: 'I am worried about not doing well in my SATS results and going to a high school when my friends aren't there'.
- Peer problems, including worries about bullying and issues around friendships: 'the girl X told me to never come into the estate again; if I do, she said she would set her pit-bull on me'.
- Family problems, including bereavement, family break-up and absence of family members: 'My dad, because I don't get to see him that much; he has been in prison twice, I get into fights a lot, I'm really worried'.
- Self-esteem issues, for example shyness and lack of confidence: 'So I can overcome my fears'.

Figure 19.1 shows an example of page 1 of the pre-therapy PSYCHLOPS Kids form, completed by a child at primary school before taking part in dramatherapy sessions. They have indicated through writing and drawing what is worrying them the most.

An interesting finding was that several children said that they had 'no problems'. The researchers wondered if this reflected a lack of understanding of the question, the impact of stigma around acknowledging problems, or a reluctance to reveal or accept that they had any problems.

At the end of the post-therapy form there is a blank sheet with the title 'Please use this space for any other comments/drawings/doodles'. Analysis of these comments and drawings showed a broad range of subjects and themes including:

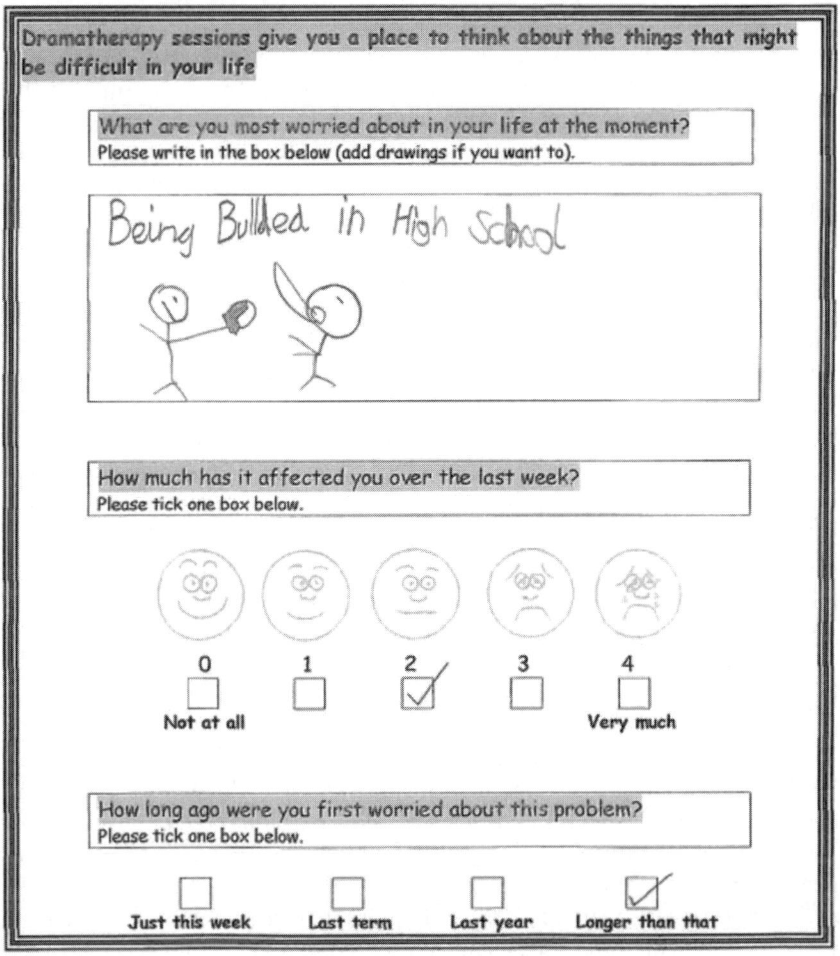

Dramatherapy sessions give you a place to think about the things that might be difficult in your life

What are you most worried about in your life at the moment?
Please write in the box below (add drawings if you want to).

Being Bullied in High School

How much has it affected you over the last week?
Please tick one box below.

0 Not at all | 1 | 2 ☑ | 3 | 4 Very much

How long ago were you first worried about this problem?
Please tick one box below.

Just this week | Last term | Last year | ☑ Longer than that

Figure 19.1 Example of completed first page of the PSYCHLOPS Kids form

> I could express myself with the other members of the group. It was the best group I ever joined.
>
> I enjoy the different activities and being able to be more confident in the class with different people. It has made me feel a lot more better [sic].
>
> Drama therapy has helped me in certain situations.

Strengths and limitations

This research represents a rigorous evaluation of dramatherapy based on a validated self-complete questionnaire. The study has created a new evaluation tool for dramatherapists to use where there was previously nothing suitable for this age group. It has helped to give a voice to children taking part in dramatherapy, which is particularly important given that documented children's view points are often absent from the evaluation of therapeutic interventions. PSYCHLOPS Kids is easy to use and evaluates the areas of concern that the children have identified for themselves. As with the adult version, these are not necessarily the ones that are highlighted in expert-selected checklist-type questionnaires (Robinson et al. 2006). It offers children the opportunity to report on the impact of their dramatherapy sessions. It also appears to be a useful starting point for the therapeutic process.

One of the main limitations of the study was the fact that the dramatherapists were reliant on the school staff both finding the time and remembering to support the children in completing PSYCHLOPS Kids before the intervention began. It also became apparent that a number of schools did not take the time to support children to complete PSYCHLOPS Kids after the dramatherapy sessions had ended, particularly if it was near the end of term. This had a significant impact on the number of completed forms. Where children were in transition to a new school, staff forgot to get the form completed before the child left. In some cases, not all the questions were completed, which meant the scores on some forms were not able to be included in the study.

Future

The research team plan in the near future to make final adjustments to PSYCHLOPS Kids, then validate it against another widely used instrument such as the SDQ. PSYCHLOPS Kids has now been finalized and is ready for use by other therapists working with children via the website psychlops.org.uk.

The researchers plan to carry out qualitative interviews with teachers, therapists and children to see what they felt about completing PSYCHLOPS Kids. They will further develop training for dramatherapists and teachers using PSYCHLOPS Kids. Further evaluation of the cross-cultural implications of the language and images used on the forms needs to be developed. The measure should enable a comparison of the efficacy of dramatherapy delivered via different modalities, such as individual versus group dramatherapy. The researchers aim also to develop further the research base for dramatherapy by working towards conducting a randomised control trial, where the main outcome measure is PSYCHLOPS Kids. However, in order to do this successfully within the voluntary sector, a research grant would be a necessity.

References

Ashworth, M. (2007) 'PSYCHLOPS – a psychometric outcome measure that is finding a niche', *Counselling & Psychotherapy Research* 7 (4), 201–202.

Ashworth, M., Evans, C. and Clement, S. (2009) 'Measuring psychological outcomes after cognitive behaviour therapy in primary care: A comparison between a new patient-generated measure "PSYCHLOPS" (Psychological Outcome Profiles) and "HADS" (Hospital Anxiety and Depression Scale)', *Journal of Mental Health* 18 (2), 169–177.

Ashworth, M., Robinson, S., Evans, C., Shepperd, M., Conolly, A. and Rowlands, G. (2007) 'What does an idiographic measure (PSYCHLOPS) tell us about the spectrum of psychological issues and scores on a nomothetic measure (CORE-OM)?' *Primary Care & Community Psychiatry* 12 (1), 7–16.

Ashworth, M., Robinson, S., Godfrey, E., Parmentier, H., Shepherd, M., Christey, J., Wright, K. and Matthews, V. (2005) 'The experiences of therapists using a new client-centred psychometric instrument, "PSYCHLOPS" ("Psychological Outcome Profiles")', *Counselling and Psychotherapy Research* 5, 37–41.

Ashworth, M., Robinson, S., Godfrey, E., Shepherd, M., Evans, C., Seed, P., Parmentier, H. and Tylee, A. (2005) 'Measuring mental health outcomes in primary care: The psychometric properties of a new patient generated outcome measure "PSYCHLOPS" ("psychological outcomes profile")', *Primary Care Mental Health* 3, 261–270.

Ashworth, M., Shepherd, M., Christey, J., Matthews, V., Wright, K., Parmentier, H., Robinson, S. and Godfrey, E. (2004) 'A client-centred psychometric instrument: The development of "PSYCHLOPS" ("Psychological Outcome Profiles")', *Counselling and Psychotherapy Research* 4 (2), 27–33.

Bakker, I.M., Terluin, B., van Marwijk, H.W., van der Windt, D.A., Rijmen, F., van Mechelen, W. and Stalman, W.A. (2007) 'A cluster-randomised trial evaluating an intervention for patients with stress-related mental disorders and sick leave in primary care', *PLoS Clin Trials* 6, e26.

Barham, M. (1999) 'Come to the edge', in A. Cattanach (ed.), *Process in the Arts Therapies*. London: Jessica Kingsley.

Cohen, J. (1988) *Statistical Power Analysis for the Behavioural Sciences*, 2nd edn. Hillsdale, NJ: Lawrence Erlbaum.

Goodman, R., Meltzer, H. and Bailey, V. (1998) 'The Strengths and Difficulties Questionnaire: A pilot study on the validity of the self-report version', *European Child and Adolescent Psychiatry* 7, 125–130.

Gowers, S.G., Harrington, R.C., Whitton, A., Lelliott, P., Wing, J., Beevor, A. and Jezzard, R. (1999) 'A Brief Scale for measuring the outcomes of emotional and behavioural disorders in children: HoNOSCA', *British Journal of Psychiatry* 174, 413–416.

Grainger, R. (1999) *Researching the Arts Therapies: A Dramatherapist's Perspective*. London: Jessica Kingsley.

Jones, P. (2007) *Drama as Therapy. Theory, Practice & Research*, 2nd edn. London: Routledge.

Jones, P. and Ramsden, E. (2011) 'Ethics, children, education and therapy: Vulnerable or empowered', in A. Campbell and P. Broadhead (eds.), *Working with Children and Young People: Ethical Debates and Practices Across Disciplines and Continents*. Oxford: Peter Lang.

Karkou, V. (ed.) (2010) *Arts Therapies in Schools – Research and Practice*. London: Jessica Kingsley.

National Institute for Health and Clinical Excellence (2008) *Schools and evidence based action: NICE recommends*. London: National Institute for Health and Clinical Excellence.

Paterson, C. (1996) 'Measuring outcomes in primary care: A patient-generated measure, MYMOP, compared to the SF-36 health survey', *British Medical Journal* 312, 1016–1020.

Payne, H. (ed.) (1993) *Handbook of Inquiry in the Arts Therapies: One River, Many Currents*. London: Jessica Kingsley.

Robinson, S., Ashworth, M., Shepherd, M. and Evans, C. (2006) 'In their own words: A narrative-based classification of clients' problems on an idiographic outcome measure for talking therapy in primary care', *Primary Care Mental Health* 4, 165–173.

Schreuders, B., van Oppen, P., van Marwijk, H.W., Smit, J.H. and Stalman, W.A. (2005) 'Frequent attenders in general practice: Problem solving treatment provided by nurses', *BMC Family Practice* 6, 42.

Verhoef, M.J., Vanderheyden, L.C., Dryden, T., Mallory, D. and Ware, M.A. (2006) 'Evaluating complementary and alternative medicine interventions: In search of appropriate patient-centred outcome measures', *BMC Complementary and Alternative Medicine* 6, 38.

20 An educational psychology service evaluation of a dramatherapy intervention for children with additional needs in primary school

Jennifer Greene

Introduction

The notion of drama in relation to many children with additional needs may seem to be inappropriate and beyond their representational capabilities or level of social understanding. However, Peter (2003) argues that educational drama can offer valuable learning opportunities to such children, particularly those with social communication difficulties. Peter advocates drama to be instrumental in developing children's understanding of representations and how to use social interactions with others to create shared meanings. He argues that dramatherapy can offer vital social play opportunities, along with the potential for exploring make-believe and narrative (how events are linked) and its relationship with text. Additionally, drama can offer a unique reflective window on children's play behaviour, providing a 'learning while doing' approach to participating more meaningfully in a social world and leading towards greater social awareness and understanding.

Dramatherapy is increasingly being delivered in groups to children and young people with autistic spectrum disorder (ASD). Jones (1996) describes a case study whereby weekly dramatherapy sessions took place over two years in a day centre for young adults with ASD. These dramatherapy sessions supported the exploration and communication of difficult or distressing situations experienced by the young adults. Conn (2007) reports that dramatherapy can be used to develop the capacity for social communication, social understanding, expression and play, in a child with social communication difficulties. Some of the skills that may be developed through dramatherapy techniques include: verbal and nonverbal communication; putting oneself in the shoes of another and appreciating the different points of view (i.e. theory of mind); exploration and practice of social situations through role play.

Context of the research

Mahoney and Perales (2003) investigated the effectiveness of a relationship-focused dramatherapy intervention on the socio-emotional well-being of 20 young children with ASD or pervasive developmental disorder. Weekly intervention sessions encouraged parents to use a responsive teaching curriculum to promote the children's socio-emotional development. The intervention resulted in increases in mothers' responsiveness and significant improvements in children's social interactions. Sherratt and Peter (2002) advocate a play-drama intervention geared specifically for those with ASD, which offers a structured approach to enabling and motivating hard-to-reach children to participate more meaningfully in a social world. They contend that enabling the children to engage in playful activity will strengthen those aspects of brain functioning necessary for more flexible thinking, with associated benefits in communication skills and greater sensitivity in social interaction, consequently converting the characteristic 'triad of impairments' (Wing and Potter 2002) into a 'triad of competencies' (Peter 2003). Both of these studies employed qualitative methods of evaluation, providing an either/or description of the process and formal or informal interviews with participants.

It is apparent that there is a valid argument to provide dramatherapy interventions for children with social communication type difficulties. To date there is no strong evidence base in terms of outcomes for these groups. However, see below and PSYCHLOPS Kids (chapter 19).

The need for a dramatherapy group in a London local authority was identified through an initial pilot project that was delivered through the National Autistic Society, funded by the local authority Children's Funding. The project's aim was to provide dramatherapy for children with additional needs, and more specifically with social, communication, emotional and behavioural needs. The two dramatherapists (Holly Harbour and Karin Kilberg) involved in this project employed the oblique approach (Dekker 1987), meaning that they worked through the art form rather than directly addressing specific 'problems' or 'difficulties'. This project promotes the aims of Every Child Matters (Department for Education and Skills 2003) to 'be healthy', 'enjoy and achieve' and 'make a positive contribution', by supporting children with additional needs to develop their social and emotional skills, self-esteem and well-being.

Aims of the intervention

Special Educational Needs Coordinators (SENCOs) in two primary schools in a London local authority were given the referral criteria and they then referred children whom they felt would benefit from the intervention. The aims of the dramatherapy group were:

- to offer a safe uninterrupted space where group members felt able to explore their feelings and emotions through creative art forms
- to encourage the members to build trust in the group, to work towards working together, listening and sharing with other group members

- to encourage development around areas of communication, socialization and imagination.

Aims of the research

The Educational Psychology Service was commissioned to evaluate the effectiveness of the dramatherapy group. The aim of the evaluation was to identify any changes in children's social behaviour and adjustment in school and the community, as a result of attending dramatherapy sessions. The commissioners expressed that the purpose of this evaluation was to address the following:

- to demonstrate the impact on the children's behaviour and skills to secure further commissioning and funding
- to provide information and feedback to parents about the usefulness of dramatherapy for their child and
- to provide feedback to the dramatherapists to improve the service being provided.

Methods

The research questions posed were:

- Is there a significant difference in social skills of the children, following group attendance over 10 weeks?
- Is there a significant difference in problem behaviour following group attendance over 10 weeks?
- Is there a significant difference in academic competence following group attendance over 10 weeks?

Research paradigm and design

The Social Skills Improvement System (SSiS) Rating Scales (Gresham and Elliott, 2008) were chosen as most appropriate due to content of questions, availability of parent, child and teacher forms and length of questionnaire. It was decided to obtain the views of parents, teachers and the child to triangulate information gathered, with the aim of providing a strong evidence base.

Context and location of research

Children were referred by SENCOs in two primary schools in the London local authority. The intervention consisted of weekly one-hour sessions for 9–10 weeks with two groups of children.

Participants

Twenty children at Key Stage 1 and 2 were selected to take part in two dramatherapy groups. Of the 20 participants, 17 were male, three were female. This is proportionate to the general population as males are four times more likely to be diagnosed with social communication difficulties than females (Roth 2010). Participants were aged from 6 to 10 years old, with the average age being 7.8 years. A parent/carer and teacher of each child also completed an SSiS. The SSiS child form was deemed by the researchers and project manager to be too long for the children (with additional needs) in this research group. A short version adapted from the original was developed; this consisted of six questions (see Table 20.1).

Data collection

Multiple sources (parent, teacher and child forms) of data were collected for the 20 participants. Not all questionnaires were returned post-group. A total of nine matched pre- and post-group child questionnaires were collected. Ten teacher-matched and eight parent-matched pre- and post-group questionnaires were collected.

Data coding and analysis

The children's names (N=20) were coded for the purpose of matching pre- and post-group information. A Likert scale was applied to the child (self-score) questionnaires. All questions were scored from 1 to 4, with 1 denoting 'not true', 2 denoting 'a little true', 3 denoting 'a lot true' and 4 denoting 'very true'. The parents' and teachers' questionnaires were scored using standard directions, and scores for each participant were entered onto SPSS® 17 for Windows (Statistical Package for the Social Sciences: version 17), a data analysis tool.

Results

Descriptive statistics were obtained for the data to enable the researcher to compare the mean and median of the pre- and post-scores. A Wilcoxon signed ranks statistical test was then used to examine whether any differences were significant or were due to chance. The Wilcoxon test was administered because the data was ordinal, non-parametric (not normally distributed) and repeated measures (pre- and post-measure). The parent, teacher and child scores were analysed separately using the Wilcoxon signed ranks test. The results are reported below.

Results of the children's scale

Results from Table 20.1 below show no difference in the overall score pre- and post-intervention ($\bar{x}$=16.6). However, some change was noted for individual questions. There was a decrease in the children's response from time 1 to time 2 on question 1 'taking turns' and question 3 'make friends easily' (T1, $\bar{x}$=3.5; T2, $\bar{x}$=2.5). There was an increase for question 4 'ask others to do things with me' (T1, $\bar{x}$=2.6; T2, $\bar{x}$=3.3), question 5 'think about how others feel' (T1, $\bar{x}$=2.7; T2, $\bar{x}$=2.9) and question 6 'stay calm when dealing with problems' (T1, $\bar{x}$=1.9; T2, $\bar{x}$=2.7). There was no change for question 2, 'show others how I feel'.

A Wilcoxon signed ranks test was carried out on the data to examine whether any differences were significant (see results in Table 20.2 below). Results demonstrate that both the 'take' domain and 'friends' domain show a significant negative difference, at the 5% level (Wilcoxon, N=9, z=–2.121, two-tailed $p<0.05$), from time 1 to time 2. This implies that the children's views of their ability to take turns and to make friends easily decreased following intervention. Results showed a significant positive difference for the 'calm' domain (Wilcoxon, N=9, z=–2.070, two-tailed $p<0.05$), from time 1 to time 2. This implies that children's views of their ability to stay calm when dealing with problems increased post-intervention.

Results of the parent's scale

An analysis was carried out to determine significant difference within the two subscales (social skills and problem behaviour) and the domains within these subscales (social skills: communication, cooperation, assertion,

Table 20.1 Child questionnaire means pre- and post-intervention

		Mean ($\bar{x}$)	*Median (m)*
Question 1 'taking turns'	Time 1	3.5	4
	Time 2	2.5	2
Question 2 'show others how I feel'	Time 1	2.9	3
	Time 2	2.9	3
Question 3 'make friends easily'	Time 1	3.5	4
	Time 2	2.5	2
Question 4 'ask others to do things with me'	Time 1	2.6	2
	Time 2	3.3	4
Question 5 'think about how others feel'	Time 1	2.7	2
	Time 2	2.9	3
Question 6 'stay calm when dealing with problems'	Time 1	1.9	2
	Time 2	2.7	2
Total out of 24	Time 1	16.6	17
	Time 2	16.6	16

Table 20.2 Summary table Wilcoxon signed ranks test – child scores

	T1–T2 Take	*T1–T2 Feel*	*T1–T2 Friends*	*T1–T2 Ask*	*T1–T2 Think*	*T1–T2 Calm*
Z	–2.121[a]	0.000b	–2.121[a]	–1.318[c]	–0.541[c]	–2.070[c]
Asymptotic significance (2-tailed)	***0.034***	***1.000***	***0.034***	0.187	0.589	***0.038***

T1 – time 1; T2 – time 2; Take – taking turns; Feel – show others how I feel; Friends – make friends easily; Ask – ask other to do things with me; Think – think about how others feel; Calm – stay calm when dealing with problems.
[a] Based on positive ranks. [b] The sum of negative ranks equals the sum of positive ranks. [c] Based on negative ranks.
Scores in bold italic demonstrate significant change.

Table 20.3 Subscales standard score means

Subscale		*Mean ($\bar{x}$)*	*Median (m)*
Social skills	Pre	79.9	77.5
	Post	85.4	82.5
Problem behaviour	Pre	127.6	126
	Post	80.8	85

responsibility, empathy, engagement and self control) (problem behaviour: externalizing and internalizing).

Mean scores, shown in Table 20.3 above, demonstrated a noted increase in social skills from $\bar{x}$=79.9 to $\bar{x}$=85.4 and a decrease in problem behaviour from $\bar{x}$=127.6 to $\bar{x}$=80.8. A Wilcoxon signed ranks test was carried out to determine significant difference in these relationships; results are shown in Table 20.4 below.

Results of the Wilcoxon signed ranks test showed a significant decrease in scores for the problem behaviour subscale (Wilcoxon, N=8, z=–2.805, two-tailed p=0.05); this implies that parents reported a significant reduction in problem behaviour post-intervention.

A Wilcoxon signed ranks test was also carried out on individual domains within the social skills and problem behaviour subscales. Results are shown in Table 20.5 below. These results demonstrated a significant positive difference for the 'Empathy' domain (Wilcoxon, N=8, z=–2.136, two-tailed $p<0.05$) from time 1 to time 2, which implied parents report an increase in the child's empathy post-intervention. Results showed a significant negative difference for 'Externalizing behaviour' (Wilcoxon, N=8, z=–2.132, two-tailed $p<0.05$) from time 1 to time 2, which implies parents report a significant decrease in externalizing behaviour post-intervention.

Table 20.4 Summary table Wilcoxon signed ranks test – parent subscales

	Pre – post social skills	*Pre – post problem behaviour*
Z	–1.125[a]	–2.805[b]
Asymptotic significance (2-tailed)	0.260	0.005

[a] Based on positive ranks. [b] The sum of negative ranks equals the sum of positive ranks.

Results of teachers scale

Results, shown in Table 20.6, for the teachers' scores did not report any significant difference. Results for the domain 'Empathy' showed no significant change from time 1 to time 2 (Wilcoxon, N=10, z=0.000, two-tailed p=1.0). Results are discussed in further detail in the next section.

Summary of findings

- Within the *social skills* domain, both teachers and children reported no significant change. However, parents reported an improvement in their child's ability to show empathy towards others.
- Within the *problem behaviour* domain, children reported a noted improvement in their ability to 'stay calm when dealing with problem situations' following intervention. Parents reported a decrease in problem behaviour, with particular difference noted in externalizing behaviours (i.e. being verbally or physically aggressive, failing to control temper, and arguing); this is in agreement with the child's self-report.
- There was no significant difference in the academic competence domain, as reported by teachers.

Discussion

In the parent scores a significant positive difference in empathy from pre- to post-group demonstrated that parents perceived their child to have shown increased signs of empathy. A significant decrease was observed between time 1 to time 2 (negative relationship) for the problem behaviour subscale (internalizing and externalizing behaviour), with particular significance for externalizing behaviour (being verbally or physically aggressive, failing to control temper, and arguing). This result may imply that parents perceived less problem behaviours post-intervention. This finding is in agreement with the child's self-report of an increased ability to stay calm when dealing with problems.

Table 20.5 Summary table Wilcoxon signed ranks test – parent scores

	T1–T2 Comm	*T1–T2 Coop*	*T1–T2 Ass*	*T1–T2 Resp*	*T1–T2 Emp*	*T2–T2 Eng*	*T1–T2 SC*	*T1–T2 Ext*	*T1–T2 Int*
Z	–1.089[a]	–0.680[a]	–0.634[a]	–1.272[a]	–2.136[a]	–0.105[a]	–0.984[a]	–2.132[b]	–1.529[b]
Asymptotic significance (2-tailed)	0.276	0.496	0.526	0.203	***0.033***	0.916	0.325	***0.033***	0.126

T1 – time 1; T2 – time 2; Ass – assertion; Comm – communication; Coop – cooperation; Emp – empathy; Eng – engagement; Ext – externalizing behaviour; Resp – responsibility; SC – self-control; Int – internalizing behaviour.
[a] Based on negative ranks. [b] Based on positive ranks.
Scores in bold italic demonstrate significant change.

Table 20.6 Summary table Wilcoxon signed ranks test – teacher scores

	T1–T2 Comm	*T1–T2 Coop*	*T1–T2 Ass*	*T1–T2 Resp*	*T1–T2 Emp*	*T1–T2 Eng*	*T1–T2 SC*	*T1–T2 PBsub*	*T1–T2 Ext*	*T1–T2 Int*	*T1–T2 ACsub*
Z	–1.071(a)	–0.712[a]	–0.299[a]	–0.060[a]	0.000b	–0.905[a]	–0.365[a]	–1.125[c]	–1.355[c]	–0.210[c]	–0.656[a]
Asymptotic significance (2-tailed)	0.284	0.476	0.765	0.952	***1.000***	0.365	0.715	0.261	0.176	0.833	0.512

T1 – time 1; T2 – time 2; ACsub – academic competence subscale; Ass – assertion; Comm – communication; Coop – cooperation; Emp – empathy; Eng – engagement; Ext – externalizing behaviour; Int – internalizing behaviour; PBsub – problem behaviour subscale; Resp – responsibility ; SC – self-control.
Scores in bold italic demonstrate significant change.

[a] Based on negative ranks. [b] The sum of negative ranks equals the sum of positive ranks. [c] Based on positive ranks.

The results of the children's questionnaire showed a self-reported decrease, from 'a lot true' to 'a little true', for the concepts: 'I make friends easily' and 'I try to think about how others feel'. There may be a number of factors resulting in this change. Due to the nature and range of needs of the children, researchers cannot make a judgement about the children's understanding and response to the questions reliably, as the questionnaires were completed with the help of a teacher. In addition, it may be difficult for some of the children with social and communication-type difficulties to self-reflect on the above concepts (i.e. 'I make friends easily'). Moreover, an additional possibility may be that the dramatherapy sessions developed the children's understanding and awareness of their behaviour towards others, therefore the children were more aware of their interactions post-group. This may account for the decrease in their self-reported behaviour. The children's scores showed a significant difference in self-reported ability to 'stay calm when dealing with a problem' from time 1 to time 2. This result may be more reliable than the concepts above because it is a more physiological response and is possibly easier for children to self-monitor and report.

No significant differences were found from the teacher-related questionnaire data. This lack of significance may be due to the fact that school is a controlled environment, often providing extra support to children with additional needs; therefore marked difference in behaviour may not be apparent over a ten-week period. Furthermore, a ten-week period is a short time in which to make a marked impact on a child's behaviour so as to be noticeable to a teacher who has a class of over 20 pupils.

Most research in dramatherapy is descriptive-based and usually involves the dramatherapists' (or facilitators') observations and commentary on the group process and narratives elicited from the group or individuals (Pendzic 2003). It may be argued that due to the creative nature of dramatherapy, more scientific measures are not an appropriate form of evaluating dramatherapy groups. However, there is a need for more formative measures to be applied. Landy (2006) reports on the lack of research in dramatherapy in comparison with other creative therapies (e.g. art, dance, music and poetry therapy) and calls for more outcome-based measures to provide solid evidence for the usefulness of dramatherapy as an intervention. There appears to be a dearth of more scientifically based forms of evaluation in the field of dramatherapy and this research appears to be amongst the first in attempting a quantitative approach.

One particular difficulty associated with the evaluation of dramatherapy is the ability to identify the dramatherapy intervention alone as the sole contributor to change, as many factors including the dramatherapy can bring about change for an individual. Future research needs to consider controlling for other factors (i.e. additional interventions or groups that the child attends in school or in the community). It would also be useful to look at the content of group processes to relate these more clearly to possible expected outcomes.

Implications for this research

Continuous evaluation is needed alongside an extension of the experimental sample sizes to generalize results. The usefulness of the teacher and child form needs to be revisited and information about the group processes and feedback from the dramatherapists may be included in future research. The evaluation of this dramatherapy intervention indicates potential success. However, dramatherapy may not be reaching the full range of pupils who might benefit (e.g. withdrawn pupils and pupils with low self-esteem). It is recommended that the scope is widened when recruiting future candidates for this study. Future provision of dramatherapy might extend attendance beyond 10 weeks to help candidates' improvement in empathy and problem behaviour generalize to the school environment as well as home.

Implications for research in dramatherapy

Landy (2006) speaks of the development of dramatherapy as a practice and the need for dramatherapists to examine strengths and weaknesses of different approaches and to consider the logic and efficacy of any particular approach. He further advocated increased teaching and learning of research methods and the writing and publication of studies, in qualitative and quantitative research, case studies, outcome studies and arts-based research studies for dramatherapists. The profession is developing and different models of practice are being applied, e.g. Sue Jennings Embodiment Projection Role-EPR framework (Jennings et al. 1994). Dramatherapists need to engage in critical thinking, in research and in publication. Haythorne, Crockford and Godfrey write in this book about a recent piece of research, Psychlops Kids (chapter 19). Dramatherapists might also consider collaborating with other creative arts therapists and psychologists to provide a more formative, systematic and scientific approach to research and evaluation.

Conclusion

This study demonstrates that following ten weeks of one-hour sessions of dramatherapy, parents reported a significant improvement in children's empathy and problem behaviours. Children also reported a significant difference in their ability to stay calm when dealing with problems. Given the restricted study samples, it is currently difficult to fully ascertain the impact of the group. Additional research is therefore needed utilizing larger sample sizes and time periods, with increased focus on controls for primary factors/interventions. This evaluation is among the first of its kind in dramatherapy, and it is a step towards providing solid evidence-based support for the effectiveness of dramatherapy groups for children with social and communication-type difficulties, although it may also be used with children with different needs. Further research needs to be carried out to link theory to practice and outcome.

Acknowledgements

The author would like to thank the project manager, Robert Dyer, and the two dramatherapists, Holly Harbour and Karin Kilberg, who were extremely helpful in explaining the purpose of the dramatherapy intervention. She would also like to give special thanks to Dr Rosemary Fitzgerald, Educational Psychologist, who was involved in the initial research design and data collection.

References

Conn, C. (2007) *Using Drama with Children on the Autism Spectrum*. Brackley: Speechmark.

Dekker, K. (1987) *The Door that is a Bridge*. UK: Sesame Institute Publication.

Department for Education and Skills (DfES) (2003) *Every Child Matters*. London: HMSO.

Gresham, F.M. and Elliott, S.N. (2008). *Social Skills Improvement System. Rating Scales Manual*. Minneapolis: Pearson.

Jennings, S., Cattanach, A., Mitchell, S., Chesner, A. and Meldrum, B. (1994) *The Handbook of Dramatherapy*. London: Routledge.

Jones, P. (1996) *Drama as Therapy, Theatre as Living*. London: Routledge.

Landy, R.J. (2006) The future of drama therapy. *The Arts in Psychotherapy*, 33 (2), 135–142.

Mahoney, G. and Perales, F. (2003) Using relationship-focused intervention to enhance the social-emotional functioning of young children with autism spectrum disorders. *Topics in Early Childhood Special Education*, 23 (2), 77–89.

Pendzic, S. (2003) 6 key areas for assessment in drama therapy. *The Arts in Psychotherapy*, 30, 91–99.

Peter, M. (2003) Drama, narrative and early learning. *British Journal of Special Education*, 30 (1), 21–27.

Roth, I. (2010) *The Autism Spectrum in the 21st Century: Exploring Psychology, Biology and Practice*. UK: Open University Press.

Sherratt, D. and Peter, M. (2002) *Developing Play and Drama in Children with Autistic Spectrum Disorders*. London: David Fulton.

Wing, L. and Potter, D. (2002) The epidemiology of autism spectrum disorders: Is the prevalence rising? *Mental Retardation and Developmental Disabilities Research Reviews*, 8, 151–161.

21 Research by the British Association of Dramatherapists and literature review

Madeline Andersen-Warren

Introduction

This chapter gives information about the types of interventions that dramatherapists based in schools provide and the reported outcomes. The sources used to gather the material are reports prepared by The British Association of Dramatherapists, using data obtained from surveys and questionnaires and a review of selected relevant dramatherapy literature. The latter is restricted to articles and chapters written in the English language and published by British publishers. Texts that meet these criteria but provide accounts of dramatherapy as practised worldwide are included; priority is given to those that include reports of evidence-based practice and/or are research-based. The emphasis of this chapter is on the services provided by dramatherapists and therapy outcomes rather than the therapy processes.

Reports by the British Association of Dramatherapists (BADth)

BADth provided information to the NHS Workforce Reviews in 2007, 2008 and 2009. The figures submitted to these reviews (which are not limited to staff employed directly by the NHS) were collated from the annual update forms sent to Full Members of the Association. These demonstrated that 152 of the respondents worked in education settings (primary, secondary and schools for pupils with specific or special needs) in full-time or part-time employment, a further 27 dramatherapists were contracted to work on a sessional basis. These figures exclude: members who were employed by an external company, charity or agency who supplied therapists to a range of workplaces; dramatherapists employed as part of a Child and Adult Mental Health Service (CAMHS) Team; those in private practice who may provide services to schools and those whose primary employment is within a particular speciality, such as after adoption services, whose work included seeing some children in a school-based setting. The 68 members who were employed by social services and the 80 members working for charities and the voluntary sector indicated that although only a small percentage of their time was dedicated to working in school settings, they maintained regular contact with teachers as well as parents or guardians.

It is often presumed that the vast majority of dramatherapists work in NHS mental health settings, but current data indicate that only 5% more dramatherapists work within the NHS than in education, education being the second largest employer. Information about whether the schools were state or otherwise funded was not requested, however it was clear the regional distribution was very uneven, as 45% of services were London-based. The evidence presented to these reviews was compiled from examples of practice templates that were created by BADth and completed by practitioners. These demonstrated that the goals and outcomes of dramatherapy met the objectives set by *Every Child Matters* and the then Government's primary initiative on Social and Emotional Aspects of Learning (SEAL). The examples relating to the latter included comments from teachers as part of the wider evaluation context; a typical observation was that the children who had engaged in group or individual dramatherapy 'became more focused during lessons and their ability to learn and communicate was enhanced'. The children asserted that they make significant improvements to their abilities to participate in emotional literacy and the social interactions required for successful and enjoyable learning. Because the above reports and their relevance to dramatherapy are covered in some detail in other chapters, specific examples are not included here.

In 2008 BADth responded to two reviews of services for children and young people: *The Bercow Review of Services for Children and Young People (10–19) with Speech and Communication Needs* and *The CAMHS Review: Next Step to Improving the Emotional Well-Being and Mental Health of Children and Young People.*

As evidence to these reports was submitted in the same year, some evidence was repeated and so a general overview is outlined below. However, before outlining the main points, it is pertinent to provide information at this juncture about the major assessment and evaluation methods used by dramatherapists to prove their work is effective. A BADth-commissioned survey of the universal or generic and profession specific assessment and evaluation methods being utilized was carried out by Winn in 2008. The subsequent report (Winn 2009) indicated that the main universal methods used for interventions with children and adolescents were: the Strengths and Difficulties Questionnaire (SDQ); Robson's (1989) Self-Esteem Questionnaire; the Health of the Nation Outcome Scales for Children and Adolescents (HoNOSCA); Soft Outcomes, Universal Learning (SOUL measures Every Child Matters' Five Outcomes); and the Briere (2005) Trauma Symptom Checklist for Young Children (TSCYC). The profession-specific measures included Jones' adaptation of The Scale of Dramatic Involvement and The Six Part Story Method devised by Lahad. Generally, the combination of universal and profession-specific methods allows the therapist to collaborate with clients to define their problem areas and strengths and formulate therapy goals in a systematic and creative way, usually in liaison with carers and other professionals. The inclusion of arts-based assessment and evaluation structures allows the dramatherapist to examine not only *what* was achieved but also *how* it was achieved. Later surveys, for example a survey distributed in 2009 to dramatherapists who work with looked-after children, indicated that Boxall Profile and Clinical Outcome Measures in Routine Evaluation for young people from 11 to 16 (YP CORE) were also in common use, along with systems devised for children and young people with specific difficulties. Client-reported outcomes were considered to be of utmost importance in dramatherapy, which is based on both humanistic and holistic philosophies of health and well-being.

The range of case examples included in the submission for the Bercow Report focused on interventions to improve speech, language and communication. Dramatherapy was a particularly effective intervention in the following areas with children who were suffering from a range of behavioural and emotional difficulties, including those with a diagnosis from the autistic spectrum:

- improving behaviour towards peers both in and out of the classroom
- increasing and maintaining cooperation with staff and peers
- improving school attendance
- becoming socially included
- correcting inappropriate behaviours, especially in relation to touch and speech
- cessation of bullying and dealing with being bullied.

The changes to behaviour were long lasting and were largely created by addressing the underlying reasons for the children's unhelpful actions by providing the appropriate dramatic structures. Grimshaw stressed the importance of addressing the former while writing about her dramatherapy practice in an educational unit for children aged between 8 and 14: 'A simple definition of the term, emotional and behavioural difficulties tells us *how* certain children behave (and that this behaviour is understood to be problematical), but it does not tell us *why* children behave in this way' (1996: 52). She continued by stating that 'Exploring the behaviour is not a means of excusing it. On the contrary . . . only by exploring and acknowledging the roots of a behavioural problem within a therapeutic context, can real and sustainable change take place' (1996: 52).

The report compiled for the CAMHS Review also included data collected by surveys and case study examples. As the remit for the review was broader, the data collected were more wide-ranging. The major cause of mental health and psychological distress for the children referred to dramatherapists during a six-month period was cited as difficulties with attachment. The other reasons for referral were:

- Trauma 13% (trauma included domestic violence in the home situation; sexual/physical abuse by adults; sexual abuse by other children including siblings; trauma prior to and during the transition to seeking asylum in Britain).
- Eating disorders 10%.
- Self-harm 9%.
- Autistic spectrum and ADHD 7%.
- Adjustment reactions 5% (grief and separation).
- Depression 5%.
- Asperger's syndrome 5%.
- Recipient of bullying 5%.
- Instigator of bullying 5%.
- Suicidal feelings 4%.
- Child with cancer 3%.
- Children born addicted to drugs 1%.
- Parent with cancer or terminal illness 1%.

The survey was designed to permit the dramatherapist to enter the reason for referral to the dramatherapy service rather than ticking preselected possible reasons. The highest reason for referral was attachment difficulties, which may well have been caused by many of the other reasons and behaviours listed above. Fifty-seven per cent of the work took place in schools, the reasons for referral being evenly distributed between schools and housing associations, settings for young offenders, GP surgeries, NHS CAMHS teams, foster care services and nursery schools, with some individuals working in specialised services such as cancer care.

Regular contact with families, carers and significant others was considered an important aspect of the therapy. Eighty-six per cent of the respondents provided regular therapy sessions or a series of therapy sessions with parents, foster or adoptive parents to help them to explore or resolve their feelings in relation to the client and/or develop different parenting strategies. Ten per cent of these included siblings and members of the extended family.

Joint working with other professionals was also viewed as an essential component of good practice. In addition to participating in multidisciplinary meetings, the dramatherapists also liaised closely with teachers, occupational therapists, social workers, speech and language therapists, nurses, midwives, health visitors, dieticians, learning mentors, psychologists, police, BEST teams and other psychotherapists. Some groups were jointly run by dramatherapists and occupational therapists, speech and language therapists, play therapists or psychologists, in order to offer the children a range of skills developed by a variety of professionals.

The comments recorded from the children specifically refer to drama and other creative forms as the most effective factors in the therapy, while comments from parents and teachers stressed the lasting improvements and the children's willingness to engage in dramatherapy.

The major conclusions drawn from the material included in the submission were:

> Dramatherapy is effective in addressing the mental health and psychological needs of children and young people. Social exclusion is an important factor in the increasing level of violence and early intervention is of vital importance.
> [Dramatherapists] work actively with families and carers who might be affected emotionally by the issues surrounding [the child's] mental health and/or psychological difficulties.
>
> (BADth 2008b: 11)

BADth played an active role in providing information for the *Arts Therapies: Art, Dance Movement, Drama: Hitting The HEAT (Health, Efficiency, and Access Treatment) Targets* (Karkou 2010). This report was produced by The Scottish Arts Therapies Forum and funded by NHS Scotland. A vignette by Smyth is based on a referral made by a school nurse and is included in the document as a dramatherapy example of fulfilling the targets. The referral for the 14-year-old boy was 'due to the level of concern at the escalating cutting of his arms with a razor blade, in addition to his mood oscillation and social withdrawal' (Smyth 2010: 16). The dramatherapy intervention combined with liaison with the school team meant that the boy was helped to 'deal with the issues he was facing without the need for referral to a higher tariff service such as psychiatry. By the end of Dramatherapy there was a marked reduction in his depressive symptoms. Prescription of drugs was avoided, positively influencing the relevant HEAT target on the reduction of anti-depressants' (2010: 52).

The research undertaken by BADth indicates that dramatherapy in schools is a growing field producing positive outcomes, however, more research is required in order to generalize the findings from the case examples.

Literature review

The focus of this review is on chapters and articles that are research-based. This means that the full spectrum of dramatherapy provision in schools is not represented here. However, the literature presents a range of research methods to investigate the effectiveness of dramatherapy. The first two examples are of group work with pupils on the autistic spectrum.

A research project funded by The Mental Health Foundation from August 2004 to September 2005 was based at Portree High School, Scotland and facilitated by Helen Scott-Danter. The research methodology was based on a hermeneutic approach using 'a variety of sources and stories, or "triangulations" ranging, in this instance, from the sessions themselves, to the use of dramatherapeutic observation and assessment tools, to a questionnaire for parents, of focus group discussions with the pupils, to a journal kept by the pupils themselves' (Scott-Danter 2006: 54).

The dramatherapy assessments used were Jones' adaptation of The Scale of Dramatic Involvement 'for measuring dramatic involvement of individuals in role-play or story-telling' (Scott-Danter 2006: 57), and Kott's 'semiotic-based assessment for the purposes of "Meaning in Dramatherapy" (an expressive inventory)' (2006: 57). These scales were used at five- or six-weekly intervals.

The group ran over 24 weeks and involved three participants with an average age of 13; the main therapy aim was 'to evaluate the impact of the dramatherapy interventions on the children's social interaction and perspective taking, i.e. their capacity to empathise with others' (2006: 55).

The evaluation showed that the pupils' social interactions and communication skills improved and their anxiety relating to their diagnosis decreased. The principal teacher commented that 'Dramatherapy is crucial in helping ASD pupils improve their communication and cooperation skills. Both parents and teachers are often forced to use a reward system to achieve cooperation. What Dramatherapy did was to achieve this cooperation on a voluntary basis. This is the kind of learning that lasts' (2006: 60).

Scott-Danter provides detailed session plans and assessment and evaluation charts of this pilot study so the research could be replicated, tested and generalized.

Miller's (2005) account of working with children with pervasive development disorders (including autistic spectrum disorder, Asperger's syndrome and Rett's disorder). Her aim was to assist the children to develop friendship skills. The dramatherapy was evaluated via questionnaires and monitoring changes from baseline skills. After ten sessions the participants and teachers recorded increased and appropriate contact with others.

Tytherleigh and Karkou also focused on the development of building relations with children on the autistic spectrum who attended a special school. They used case-study research methods and information was collected via: 'participant observation; observation of video recording sessions; observations of clients outside sessions; reflection with co-worker and clients; discussion with the class teacher and client's parents' (2010: 203).

The research, based on six sessions with two 11-year-old children, demonstrated that embodied and sensory play, drama and movement structures and dramatic games coupled with projective techniques are interventions that may help to achieve relationship-building.

Christensen (2010) provides a further example of case-study research in a school-based student support unit for students aged between 11 and 19. Her research question was 'What are the experiences and perceptions of an adolescent boy in an SSU of the contribution that dramatherapy can make regarding reintegration into a community college?' (2010: 88). The specific dramatherapy assessment methods employed were The Six Part Story Method, (Lahad 1992) and The Five Story Structure Method (Casson 2004). Six 13-year-old boys engaged in individual dramatherapy were involved with the research; the voices of the children were central to the study. Post-therapy interviews were analysed using thematic analysis methods. The chapter includes detailed material about the interventions used with one boy, with extracts from the dramatherapists' clinical notes about the reasons for and the consequences of specific interventions.

The data obtained from this study suggest that dramatherapy was an effective component of the children's partial or complete integration into school following brief focused interventions. Smyth also provides an account of brief, focused dramatherapy based in a school in Sri Lanka using single case-study research methods. The goals set were for the ten children aged between 12 and 13 to be able to engage in conflict resolution and in cooperative play. Her data were collected by using session logs, 'life-mapping diagrams, social games and group-building exercises . . . reflective diaries and personal process notes' (2010: 102). She describes her approach as 'process-orientated and holistic' and her contention is that this method helped her to 'gather naturally occurring, emergent and qualitative information' (2010: 102). A thematic analysis of the data confirmed that the therapeutic goals had been reached.

McArdle et al. (2002) report that a randomized control study that involved 136 children indicated that the dramatherapy group therapy could be effective in supporting children at risk of emotional or behavioural problems, including anxiety and depression. Dramatherapy was seen as particularly effective by both the children and teachers involved in the study, more so than by parents. Dramatherapy was more effective than the intervention used in the control group (small-group curriculum studies), with benefits remaining for one year following the groups. A further account of this study is provided by Quibell (2010), one of the authors of the 2002 article.

Narrative research into dramatherapy theory and practice has been pioneered by Jones (2007, 2010) and he provides valuable information about a range of dramatherapy interventions in a wide variety of settings.

The research culture within the dramatherapy field is developing quickly and will continue to grow, encompassing a plethora of research methods.

References

BADth (2008a) Submission to *The Bercow Review of Services for Children and Young People (10–19) with Speech and Communication Needs*. Available at: www.BADth.org.uk members' area (Accessed 16 January 2011).

BADth (2008b) Submission to *The CAMHS Review: Next Step to Improving the Emotional Well-Being and Mental Health of Children and Young People*. Available at: www.Badth.org.uk members' area (Accessed 16 January 2011).

Boxall Profile. Available at: www.Nuturegroup.org (Accessed 17 January 2011).

Briere, J. (2005) *The Trauma Symptom Checklist for Young Children – Professional Manual* Odessa: Psychological Resource, Inc.

Casson, J. (2004) *Drama, Psychotherapy and Psychosis: Dramatherapy and Psychodrama with People Who Hear Voices*. Hove: Brunner-Routledge.

Christensen, J. (2010) 'Making space inside: The experience of dramatherapy within a school-based student support unit', in V. Karkou (ed.), *Arts Therapies in Schools: Research and Practice*. London: Jessica Kingsley.

Clinical Outcome Measures: Young People. *CORE: A Decade of Development*. Available at: www.coreims.co.uk (Accessed 17 January 2011).

Grimshaw, D. (1996) 'Dramatherapy with children in an educational unit', in S. Mitchell (ed.), *Dramatherapy: Clinical Studies*. London: Jessica Kingsley.

Jones, P. (2007) *Drama as Therapy: Theory, Practice and Research, Volume 1*. Hove: Routledge.

Jones, P. (2010) *Drama as Therapy: Clinical Work and Research into Practice, Volume 2*. Hove: Routledge.

Karkou, K. (2010) *Arts Therapies: Art, Dance Movement, Drama: Hitting The HEAT Targets*. Available at: www.nhshealthquality.org (Accessed 18 January 2011).

Lahad, M. (1992) 'Story making as an assessment method for coping with stress', in S. Jennings (ed.), *Dramatherapy: Theory and Practice 2*. London: Routledge.

McArdle, P., Moseley, D., Quibel, T., Johnson, R., Allen, A., Hammal, D. and Le Couteur, A. (2002) 'School-based indicated prevention: A randomised trial of group therapy'. *Journal of Child Psychology and Psychiatry*, 43, 705–712.

Miller, C. (2005) 'Developing friendship skills with children with pervasive developmental disorders: A case study'. *Dramatherapy: Journal of British Association of Dramatherapists*, 27, 11–16.

Quibell, T. (2010) 'The searching drama of disaffection: dramatherapy groups in a whole school context', in V. Karkou (ed.), *Arts Therapies in Schools: Research and Practice*. London: Jessica Kingsley.

Robson, P. (1989) 'Development of a new self-report questionnaire to measure self-esteem'. *Psychological Medicine*, 19, 513–518.

Scott-Danter, H. (2006) 'Dramatherapy autistic spectrum, Portree High School', in *Arts, Creativity and Mental Health Initiative: Reports from four arts therapies trial services 2003–2005*. London and Scotland: Mental Health Foundation.

SDQ (Strengths and Difficulties Questionnaire). Available at: www.sdqinfo.com (Accessed 18 January 2011).

Smyth, G. (2010) 'Solution-focused brief dramatherapy group work: Working with children in mainstream education in Sri Lanka', in V. Karkou (ed.), *Arts Therapies in Schools: Research and Practice*. London: Jessica Kingsley.

Tytherleigh, L. and Karkou, V. (2010) 'Dramatherapy, autism and relationship-building', in V. Karkou (ed.), *Arts Therapies in Schools: Research and Practice*. London: Jessica Kingsley.

Winn, L. (2009) *The Use of Outcome Measures in Dramatherapy*. Available at: www.BADth.org.uk members' area (Accessed 15 January 2011).

Part V

Future possibilities

22 Educational psychology, listening to children and dramatherapy

Irvine Gersch

And therefore as a stranger give it welcome.
There are more things in heaven and earth, Horatio,
Than are dreamt of in your philosophy.
(Shakespeare, *Hamlet* Act 1: Scene V)

Introduction

This chapter explores how educational psychologists and dramatherapists might work closer together and, in particular, how some developing work in the field of listening to children might provide profitable areas of shared activity and cross-fertilization of ideas. The chapter begins by outlining briefly the role of educational psychologists, and then reviews some of the author's work on listening to children, culminating in the most recent work on spiritual listening. The next section focuses upon the views of educational psychologists about dramatherapy, showing the current limited knowledge and awareness, before going on to suggest a new model for future working.

The role of the educational psychologist

Educational psychologists work with children and young people, parents and teachers, as well as other professionals to promote the emotional, social and educational development of children and young people. They work at a variety of levels, offering direct work with children and young people, work with parents, advice and consultation to schools, as well as supervision, systems work or projects in schools, research and training. They help to develop local authority policy in areas of special needs and child development. They also work with other agencies in the community.

A major Department for Education and Employment (DfEE) report on educational psychology describes the key aim or purpose of the contribution of educational psychologists as 'to promote child development and learning through the application of psychology by working with individual and groups of children, teachers and other adults in schools, families, other LEA officers, health and social services and other agencies' (2000a: 5). This report identified the core areas of activity as being early years work, work with schools and multi-agency work.

Since that time and further reports (e.g. Woods et al. 2006), as well as the commencement of the Every Child Matters agenda, and other structural changes in local authorities, it could be argued that the role of the educational psychologist has widened, particularly in the areas of multi-agency and community work.

A large measure of this much varied work is within schools and Early Years settings, working with children and young people at the individual level, through assessments and intervention. It is also fair to say that the extent of each of these activities actually delivered does in fact vary, from area to area, and even within educational psychology services.

That said, educational psychologists are required to carry out statutory assessments under the 1996 Education Act (DfEE 1996) and to provide formal psychological advice for those children and young people whose special educational needs are being formally assessed. However, many educational psychologists wish to devote much more time to intervention and therapeutic work (DfEE 2000b). This is echoed in schools, where many members of staff perceive unmet needs of children with emotional issues and look to educational psychologists to provide therapeutic advice and direct work with these children.

The training of educational psychologists has recently been extended from one to three years, full time, and raised from Masters to Doctoral level, to ensure comprehensive coverage of all of those areas that have been mentioned. At the University of East London (where the author acted as programme director for this programme until 2009), as in many, though not all institutions that provide such training, this course is entitled a 'Doctorate in Educational and Child Psychology'.

Listening to children

Since 1984 the author has been involved in developing ideas to increase the participation and involvement of children in their assessments, and exploring ways and techniques of listening to children more effectively and eliciting and valuing their views. The first project, carried out as early as 1985, was the development of the Child's Report, for children in care of the local authority. This led to the Student Report (1994), the Excluded Pupils' Report (1994) and Student Advice (2000).

These devices were developed purely to offer the child the opportunity to express his or her own views, formally and emphatically, and to ensure that such views were afforded an important and meaningful place in the assessment process.

Details are provided in a series of publications (Gersch and Cutting 1985; Scherer, Gersch and Fry 1990; Gersch and Holgate 1991; Gersch 1992;

Gersch, Holgate and Sigston 1993; Gersch and Nolan 1994; Gersch and Gersch 1995; Gersch 1995; Gersch, Pratt, Nolan and Hooper, 1996; Gersch 1996a; Gersch 2001a).

The case was made that such involvement had three main elements: pragmatic, moral and legal. In addition, it was helpful for teachers in providing feedback and it created a listening ethos in schools (Gersch 1996a).

The Student Report, which is a report completed by children and young people themselves and which over the years has been revised and modified in the light of student feedback, has eight major headings, which are:

- Background
- School
- Special needs
- Friends
- Out of school
- Feelings
- The future
- Anything else.

This report has been translated into community languages, modified and abbreviated for use within the statutory assessment procedure and for use as the student's contribution to their statutory assessment.

It is fair to say that during the past 25 years, there has been an increased acceptance and valuing of listening to children's views in education, with many examples seen of Pupil Councils in schools, and pupil feedback being sought.

The fact that children's views have to be ascertained for Special Educational Needs (SEN) assessments in accordance with the SEN Code of Practice (Department for Education and Skills 2001) and when legal appeals are lodged to the SEN and Disability Tribunal, as well as the creation of the post of Children's Commissioner (known as the Children's Ombudsman), all testify to this trend.

The United Nations Convention on the Rights of the Child, which was signed by the UK and came into force in 1990, states that:

> States Parties shall assure to the child who is capable of forming his or her own views the right to express those views freely in all matters affecting the child, the views of the child being given due weight in accordance with the age and maturity of the child.
>
> For this purpose, the child shall in particular be provided the opportunity to be heard in any judicial and administrative proceedings affecting the child, either directly, or through a representative or an appropriate body, in a manner consistent with the procedural rules of national law.
>
> (United Nations Convention 1989: Article 12)

In the UK this is enshrined in SEN Legislation in the SEN Code of Practice (Department for Education and Skills 2001), the Education Act (DfEE 1996) and the Children Act (Department of Health 1989) and appears throughout the thinking in the Every Child Matters agenda.

The issue of listening to children is not without its challenges, critique and dilemmas. Listening is a two-way process and children do need to learn effective ways of expressing their ideas to adults. Children do not always have the experience, maturity or wisdom to make all the decisions required of them, nor can they necessarily know what is best for them. In addition, for a variety of reasons, children are not always truthful and, as with all humans, their memories and recall abilities are open to error. Consequently, I would argue that it is always necessary for adults to adopt their proper adult, parental and teacher role, to involve children and young people to a level that is appropriate for the decision and, of course, reflecting the young person's maturity, understanding and capability.

Having said that, I would argue that it would always be beneficial to learn about and understand the child's perspective, feelings and ideas. In my experience, adults have been positively surprised by the sensible and important ideas expressed by even very young children and those with profound special needs.

What is needed are ways of eliciting the child's views when these may be difficult to obtain, for example, with children who are unable to express their true feeling or anxieties, or when those with special educational needs have to cross real barriers to physical communication. In my view, these are challenges that need to be overcome, rather than permanent limitations, and require creative responses, with adults developing skills of listening deeply and, of course, taking the time needed to facilitate effective and meaningful communication.

These are complex issues that indicate that the degree of children's involvement in their assessment and education lies along a continuum, from minimal child involvement and participation to maximum involvement and participation. I would argue that a desirable aim is for us to seek to increase the child and young person's involvement, as far as possible.

This work has led to a project exploring ways of listening to children at a deeper level, which I have termed 'spiritual listening', discussed in the next section.

Spiritual listening

The author's work on listening to children has led to an attempt at this stage to explore the deeper views and thoughts that children might be able to voice. The work has been informed by early philosophers, such as Plato, Socrates and others, as well as more recent work by Frankl (1984), Goleman (1995) and Zohar and Marshall (2001), and it has been developed with a project team at UEL (Gersch, Dowling, Panagiotaki and Potton 2008).

This work has led to the development of a 'Spiritual Listening Tool' (Lipscomb and Gersch 2011; Gersch et al. 2008), for psychologists to use when working with children and young people in order to elicit the child's perspective about their deeper views and ideas.

Taking the definition of spirit as an animating or vital drive, Zohar and Marshall (2001) argued that humans are essentially driven by a longing to find meaning and purpose to their lives, and these meanings actually drive and define people and create a sense of worth.

A small group of children were asked metaphysical or deep questions, such as 'What makes you happy, or unhappy? What makes for a happy or an unhappy life? How do you think the world was made? Have you heard of the word "soul"? Do you think we are living in the world for a reason? Is it possible for people to live in peace without war and conflict? Do you think there is life on other planets? Do you think our lives are influenced by fate and destiny? Do you think these issues affect how children behave or learn?'

What emerged from the actual answers given by a small group of children was that children were very well able to reply sensibly and clearly to these questions, and that they felt them to be important in influencing behaviour and learning. The detailed answers are to be found in a full paper (Gersch et al. 2008). Of note was the fact that when they spoke of what made them happy or sad, they focused predominantly on relationships and non-material things.

The authors felt that this small and limited pilot should be followed by further studies. It is interesting to note that others working in education have begun to focus on wellbeing in schools and to use the teachings of philosophy when working with children in order to extend thinking skills, to encourage curiosity and questioning, and to promote emotional development and skills related to moral judgement. One such example is a programme produced by White (2001) entitled 'Philosophy for Kids'.

The next section will focus upon partnership possibilities between educational psychologists and dramatherapists.

Partnership possibilities between educational psychologists and dramatherapists

Our own research at UEL on arts therapies (Gersch and Goncalves 2006) has shown that despite the fact that educational psychologists and dramatherapists work in the same domain, albeit using different methods and theoretical frameworks, and despite having shared professional interests, the link between educational psychologists and dramatherapists is, in reality, very limited indeed in local authorities, where the majority of educational psychologists are employed.

Of a small sample of 22 educational psychologists asked about arts therapists, 73% knew about their role, 55% knew about the work they undertook, 41% had met an arts therapist (i.e. art therapist, music therapist, dramatherapist), but only 5% had any plans for joint work or intervention with any type of arts therapist. One would therefore surmise that this would involve even fewer dramatherapists.

However, and this is a key point, 59% of educational psychologists who were sampled thought that it would be important to work jointly with such arts therapists. Further, most of these educational psychologists rated highly the work of arts therapists, they believed this work to be very beneficial for children, and they wanted to learn more about the role and work of all arts therapists during their own training.

During an informal discussion with a colleague dramatherapist (Goodman 2010), it was explained that the emphasis of dramatherapy is, or should be, as much about *hearing* as listening. In dramatherapy, close attention is paid to things that are being said, as well as those things that are being left unsaid, or are difficult to express, and most importantly, the meaning of what is being told. The dramatherapist will be alive to the nuances of such communication, as well as recurrent and key themes, all the time exploring ways of working with interpretations that help the client make sense of their life circumstances and gain insight into them.

According to Goodman, such hearing and listening should be *active, respectful, containing, trusting* and *follow the journey and narrative of the person being assisted.* She further argues that the quality of this hearing and listening is fundamental to the establishment of a secure therapeutic relationship, in which the child can feel truly 'heard' and understood. It is within the safety of such a relationship that the child's story or narrative can be told and worked with. Through the use of dramatherapy techniques, such as games, story telling and story making, movement and role play, underlying themes may be expressed and explored metaphorically, offering opportunities to gain insight into troubling issues. In so doing, the client is helped to find new ways of relating and dealing with personal difficulties. Indeed, working through stories, acting, role-play, games, and other dramatherapy activities can have a major impact upon the client's life, and the way they view and understand things.

Goodman has explained that, in her experience, the impact of skilled witnessing itself should not be underestimated. Thus, in dramatherapy, clients are invited to both express their deep feelings and ideas, and through careful listening, hearing and witnessing, they are enabled to work though deep thoughts and connections. The aims are to promote personal growth and self-esteem as well as to address any particular difficulties, issues or challenges that clients might bring.

Indeed, one could argue that the essence of dramatherapy, apart from gaining a deeper understanding of the child's inner world, through establishing a safe, containing, and trusted therapeutic relationship, is to enable the child's growth through the use of these ideas. Using a variety of dramatic activities, which may include movement, improvisation, storytelling, the use of metaphors and role play, communication appears to be possible at a deep level between client and therapist.

Sessions may be individual or with small groups. They essentially follow a series of segments, from Introduction to Main Content, to Closing Stages, with a variety of combinations in any particular context and setting.

The aims of dramatherapy are highly consonant with those of educational psychology. Importantly, our work on listening to children specifically dovetails perfectly with the work of dramatherapy and seems to me to be an example of a direct link that has not been fully utilized for the benefit of children with special or additional needs, or even those facing temporary life challenges. I am sure that there are other such mutually consonant projects and areas worthy of joint research, development and practice.

Working in a forensic, psychiatric, secure hospital, Goodman has noted from her own work and experience that the roots of psychological difficulties often seem to stem back to childhood, family dysfunction and insecure attachments, which have interfered with healthy emotional development. She has often speculated whether intervention at an earlier stage, when problems are first evident, could provide a powerful role in preventing problems later in life.

Some ideas for future action

So, how could this link be developed and promoted, in practice?

Some ideas that have been discussed elsewhere, and to which the reader is referred, are raised in Gersch (2001b). These include possible ways of explaining and 'selling' dramatherapy, identifying potential customers, carrying out market research, identifying key decision makers in the school, explaining the role and benefits and limitations of dramatherapy, pricing, contracting, and offering an evaluated time-limited pilot scheme.

In addition, the following ideas could be considered:

- Educational psychologists should learn more about the work of dramatherapists during their initial training and through continuing professional development and training.
- Dramatherapists should be invited to find out more about the work of educational psychologists, at national conferences, through publications and other communications and through their training.
- In particular geographical localities, dramatherapists and educational psychologists might well introduce themselves to each other, seek each other out, and discuss ways for potential working together, perhaps through assessment, treatment/interventions and joint training offered to schools and CAMHS services. This does not necessarily mean that educational psychologists and dramatherapists have to work together

contemporaneously or in the same place or location on cases (although this would be an interesting idea and could take place if circumstances permit). Rather, these professionals, who have much in common, could perhaps plan their work together, review their progress together and perhaps arrange joint peer supervision and sharing.

- At policy level, dramatherapists and educational psychologists should perhaps discuss their work with policy makers, e.g. Local Authority Directors of Services and with central government, when opportunities arise. They should continue to respond emphatically to government consultations. (It is of note that the new Coalition Government published a Green Paper *Support and aspiration: A new approach to special educational needs and disability* in March 2011; Department for Education 2011.)
- Local scoping and local responses are particularly important in developing this link, because dramatherapists are not available throughout the country, and because access is complex and dependant upon local circumstances, and even the funding of dramatherapy is both variable and not always clear. For example, some CAMHS services and schools may employ dramatherapists, but most do not. Parents may be able to buy such therapy for their children, if they were aware of that option but, in my experience, most do not.
- It may be that dramatherapists could offer a service to a group of schools, and indeed, it would appear from the latest White Paper (Department for Education 2010) that schools will be able to afford even greater choice over the services they commission, certainly offering new opportunities for dramatherapists. In this regard, it is vital to gain an insight into the feelings and perceptions of teachers themselves (Gersch 1996b).
- Dramatherapists could also be involved in the recent government initiative called 'Team around the Child', whereby local teams are set up to provide comprehensive packages for children with additional and special needs. Local exploration would be needed to examine how to become involved in such a process.
- The setting up of a small task force of both dramatherapists and educational psychologists would be useful in order to explore how further links could be put into practice and promoted. This might be set up formally under the auspices of the British Psychological Society, the Association of Educational Psychologists and the British Association of Dramatherapists. It could be extended to include representatives of other arts therapies and it could perhaps include representatives from the Health Professionals Council.
- I am aware that a number of dramatherapists on the executive of the British Association of Dramatherapists are working hard to ensure representation on key national governmental sub-committees, and I feel sure that such work will continue to raise the profile and promote

the work of dramatherapists. This work is clearly important, necessary and worthwhile.

Conclusions

It is the underlying thesis of this chapter, and indeed this book, that dramatherapy is something of an untold story in respect of allied professionals in schools and among the public, and that it is important to pick up the waves of energy of new schools' freedoms, legislation, the new Green Paper, and listening to children. In addition, there are major opportunities for joint work with educational psychologists and others to promote and publicize this exciting, innovative and important professional approach to working deeply with children. Hopefully, this will have a positive impact for change on the lives of children and young people, and those of their families and be of help to schools. Most specifically, it has been argued that there is significant scope for developing the relationship between the two professional groups of dramatherapy and educational psychology.

References

Department for Education and Employment (1996) *Education Act*. London: DfEE Publications.

Department for Education and Employment (2000a) *Educational Psychology Services (England). Current Role, Good Practice and Future Directions. Report of the Working Group*. Nottingham: DfEE Publications.

Department for Education and Employment (2000b) *Educational Psychology Services (England). Current Role, Good Practice and Future Directions. Research Report*. Nottingham: DfEE Publications.

Department for Education and Skills (2001) *SEN Code of Practice on the Identification and Assessment of Special Educational Needs*. London: DfES.

Department for Education (2010) *The Schools White Paper: The Importance of Teaching*. London: TSO.

Department for Education (2011) *Support and aspiration: A new approach to special educational needs and disability – A consultation*. CM 8027. London: TSO

Department of Health (1989) *The Children Act*. London: HMSO.

Frankl, V. (2004) *Man's Search for Meaning*. London: Random House.

Gersch, I.S. (1992) 'Pupil involvement in assessment', in T. Cline (ed.), *The Assessment of Special Educational Needs: International Perspectives*. London: Routledge.

Gersch, I.S. (1995) 'The Pupil's View'. *Briefing Pack for Schools on the Code of Practice*. National Children's Bureau in association with the DfE.

Gersch, I.S. (1996a) 'Involving children in assessment: Creating a listening ethos'. *DECP Educational and Child Psychology*, 13 (2), 3–40.

Gersch, I.S. (1996b) 'Teachers are people too. Support for learning: special issue on children with emotional and/or behavioural difficulties'. *British Journal of Learning Support*, 11 (4), 165–169.

Gersch, I.S. (2001a) 'Listening to children. In practice and policy in schools', in J.

Wearmouth (ed.), *Special Educational Provision in the Context of Inclusion*. London: David Fulton.

Gersch, I.S. (2001b) 'Dramatherapy in education: opportunities for the future – a view from the outside'. *Dramatherapy, Special 'Education' Edition*, 23 (1), 4–8.

Gersch, I.S. and Cutting, M.C. (1985) 'The Child's Report'. *Educational Psychology in Practice*, 1 (2), 63–69.

Gersch, I.S. and Gersch, B. (1995) 'Supporting advocacy and self-advocacy: the role of allied professions in advocacy, self-advocacy and special needs', in P. Garner and S. Sandow (eds.), *Advocacy, Self Advocacy and Special Needs*. London: David Fulton.

Gersch, I.S. and Holgate, A. (1991) *The Student Report*. London Borough of Waltham Forest.

Gersch, I.S. and Nolan, A. (1994) 'Exclusions: What the pupils think'. *Educational Psychology in Practice*, 10 (1), 35–45.

Gersch, I.S. and Sao Joao Goncalves, S. (2006) 'Creative arts and educational psychology: Let's get together'. *International Journal of Art Therapy*, 11 (1), 22–32.

Gersch, I.S., Dowling, F., Panagiotaki, G. and Potton, A. (2008) 'Children's views of spiritual and metaphysical concepts: a new dimension to educational psychology practice'. *Educational Psychology in Practice*, 24 (3), 225–236.

Gersch, I.S., Holgate, A. and Sigston, A. (1993) 'Valuing the child's perspective: a revised student report and other practical initiatives'. *Educational Psychology in Practice*, 9 (1), 36–45.

Gersch, I.S. with Pratt, G., Nolan, A. and Hooper, S. (1996) 'Listening to children: The educational context', in Upton, G. et al. (eds.), *The Voice of the Child: A Handbook for Professionals*. London: Falmer Press.

Goleman, D. (1995) *Emotional Intelligence*. New York: Bantum Books.

Goodman, R. (2010) Personal communication, 27 December.

Lipscomb, A. and Gersch, I.S. (2011) 'The development of a spiritual listening tool for educational psychology practice'. *Educational Psychology in Practice*, forthcoming.

Scherer, M., Gersch, I.S. and Fry, L. (1990) *Meeting Disruptive Behaviour: Assessment, Intervention and Partnership*. London: Macmillan Education.

United Nations Convention on the Rights of the Child (1989) Available at: http://www2.ohchr.org/english/law/crc.htm (Accessed 1 January 2010).

White, D.A. (2001) *Philosophy for Kids: 40 Fun Questions That Help You Wonder About Everything*. Texas: Prufrock Press.

Woods, K.A., Farrell, P.T., Lewis, S., Squires, G., Rooney, S. and O'Connor, M. (2006) *Review of the Function and Contribution of Educational Psychologists in Light of the 'Every Child Matters Agenda'*. Research Report 792 DFES.

Zohar, D. and Marshall, I. (2001) *Spiritual Intelligence: The Ultimate Intelligence*. London: Bloomsbury.

23 A model of emotional support in primary schools

Brenda Meldrum

Introduction

There are three main ways – not necessarily mutually exclusive – of setting up emotional support for children in schools:

- the first way is when the school buys-in a school-based external agency that provides counsellors/therapists and their own manager;
- the second way is to employ dramatherapists, other arts therapists and play therapists and/or school counsellors to work with children who are of concern;
- the third way is for the school to develop an emotional support programme itself, using school staff who receive appropriate training.

In this chapter, I address the second way of giving schoolchildren emotional support. I concentrate on the profession of dramatherapy, but I should stress that other arts therapists, play therapists and school counsellors might also be considered for this work. Dramatherapists use drama, music, dance, creative materials and play as the therapeutic media to help children's emotional expression through metaphor, symbols and stories; these processes are largely non-verbal and playful, which is the way that children understand and communicate.

Communication develops within relationships. Young children especially are much more in tune with the non-verbal messages in adults' communication than in the meaning of the words; actions really speak louder than words, because the non-verbal gesture or facial expression or tone of voice carries the emotional message that may well conflict with our words. Human beings are highly attuned to the non-verbal aspect of communication and are constantly monitoring the emotional states of others through their body language. The infant brain is geared to recognize, process and remember emotional states, including the recognition of the affective content of people's facial expressions, their tone of voice and the quality of their movements – whether abrupt or smooth. And it is evident that the ability to manage our emotional reactions to others and to events is a skill learned in early childhood within the primary attachment relationship between adult and child (Bowlby 1988). Indeed, attachment behaviours are non-verbal. Positive emotions, such as the pleasure of playing with the responsive parent, help children approach, pay attention for longer periods, find huge enjoyment in the interaction, and learn the way we both manage our emotions and understand how to make social relations. Emotions, expressed in joint play, function to help the child adapt to and coordinate with other people and manage behaviour. They operate as central organizing processes within the brain and give our memories and thoughts colour, meaning and value.

Howe (2005), in a development of Bowlby's theory, defines attachment *as the theory of emotional regulation*. He observes that the secure mother not only continuously regulates her child's level of arousal, but also introduces the child to the world outside the dyad – other family members, and also to emotions and feelings, thoughts and objects and, above all, to the importance of relationships and other people. Furthermore, it is these behaviours that cement the relationship of carer and infant, allowing an engagement with another mind, thus beginning the development of self through the relationship with another human being and her mind (Siegel and Hartzell 2003). Thus, the infant is born predisposed to be social and with a repertoire of behaviours designed to protect him on the one hand and to form relationships through which he develops his identity – his *self* – on the other hand. This self is forged through the mind of the person who cares for him or her: as Sue Gerhardt says so succinctly, 'the baby is an interactive project, not a self-powered one' (2004: 18).

The dramatherapy profession has been protected since 1997, when 'Dramatherapy' was registered with the Health Professionals Council (HPC) within the 'Arts Therapists' section. Thus, only those professionals who are registered with HPC may call themselves 'dramatherapists'. Employers may check lists of registered dramatherapists with the British Association of Dramatherapists as well as HPC registers. In my view, dramatherapists who have had training in working with children and also, by definition, play therapists, are in a better position than those who use the talking therapies to communicate with children and young people because they are using media that children can understand. Working as they do through their art form, dramatherapists use symbolic means of communication through the creative expression of their medium. Through the use of metaphor and symbols children can safely explore the emotional impact of their experience and tell the story through the drama, the collage or picture and through the play.

In this chapter, I look at the ways schools can set up therapeutic support in school using a dramatherapist who can work with children one-to-one and also in small groups. I itemize what I think needs to be done to set up a therapeutic project, and its management; I propose some reasons that a child may need therapeutic support and I give my suggestions for a referral process, together with referral forms as appendices.

How does the process start?

What usually happens is that head teachers recognize that there is a number of children in school whose behaviour is of concern to staff. Some children may be unable to settle and they disrupt others, some may find it hard to make friends because they hit out at other children, some may be struggling with their emotional reactions to life and family events such as conflict and parental separation; others may seem unhappy and withdrawn because they are not loved, some because their granny has died. Staff recognize that the principal need is for someone to listen and take time with these troubled children in order that they can share problems or just be with a warm, reliable person who is non-judgemental, caring and playful. At this point, decisions will be made as to whether to choose an external agency that will bring in their own management staff and volunteer and trainee counsellors, or to employ therapists or counsellors, or to keep the provision entirely school-based by training their own staff to deliver the emotional support.

Whichever is chosen, a holistic approach and a plan must be devised. In this chapter, we assume that the school decides to employ a dramatherapist.

Setting up an in-school project to give emotional support to children

In order to do this effectively, there are several prerequisites:

- *Support from the senior management team* is crucial. An emotional support project requires leadership from the top and encouragement for teaching staff, some of whom may be cynical about the efficacy of the process.
- *Consultation and education of school staff*: it is important for the success of the programme that the school staff support the work, through Staff In-Service Training (INSET) and discussion in school.
- An appointment of a *project coordinator* is essential. This is a lead person who coordinates the dramatherapist (and other support workers), who processes the referrals and manages the project under the senior management team. She should have some standing within school – for example, as the inclusion manager or the special education needs manager; thus, she will be both a trained teacher and will have received training in supporting the emotional welfare of children.
- *Recruitment of a qualified dramatherapist*, who is HPC-registered and who has received training in working therapeutically with children. The dramatherapist is given dedicated time to work one-to-one with children in a safe and secure space.
- All workers in school, including the dramatherapist, need to have had an *advanced Criminal Records Bureau* clearance before they start work.
- The dramatherapist needs *professional indemnity insurance*, as the

school's insurance may not cover the therapeutic work.

- Regular *weekly supervision* of the dramatherapist's casework by the project coordinator.
- The dramatherapist also needs to have *regular clinical supervision* by a supervisor trained in working with children.

The management of the project

There is a number of decisions that need to be made about:

- The children and the level of difficulty.
- The referral process.
- The length of the dramatherapy contract: the number of sessions.
- The secure and appropriate space for the work to take place.
- The resources and play materials needed in the therapy room.
- The timetabling of the sessions.

The children and the level of difficulty

There is currently a 4-tier widely recognized level of service in the mental health field emanating from the Child and Adolescent Mental Health Service (CAMHS). If the school goes for the *third* option and is employing its own trained staff, then these listening supporters are working at CAMHS Tier 1, which *Children and Young People in Mind: The Final Report of the National CAMHS Review* (Department for Education, 2008) describe as:

> Tier 1: CAMHS at this level are provided by practitioners who are not mental health specialists working in universal services; this includes GPs, health visitors, school nurses, teachers, social workers, youth justice workers, voluntary agencies. Practitioners will be able to offer general advice and treatment for less severe problems, contribute towards mental health promotion, identify problems early in their development and refer to more specialist services.

In the second option, the dramatherapist will be working at CAMHS Tier 2 as well as Tier 1, which enables them to take on more complex cases. All issues can be seen through the lens of attachment, as I argue in chapter 4, and in the vignettes that follow I give some reasons why children may be having difficulties in school and are in need of one-to-one emotional support:

- Children who have emotional difficulties that may arise from home: for example, *Joe's mother – a single parent – has a new baby and he becomes over-protective of his mother and finds it hard to leave her, and is tearful.*

- Children who have friendship difficulties and conflicts with peers: for example, *Sue is always falling out with one or two particular friends at school. She is continually quarrelling with them and then making friends with them again. Her school work is affected.*
- Children who need help communicating with staff and peers: for example, *Tom, an isolated, withdrawn boy whom no-one misses when he is not there, drifts in and out of friendships; when teams and groups are formed, he is always the last to be chosen.*
- Children who need help in seeing how their behaviour affects their communication with others: for example, *Gerry is the class clown; he is provocative with the teaching staff and always has an appreciative audience in the classroom. He takes up a lot of teaching time.*
- Children who are angry and confrontational: for example, *Usman whose fears and unhappiness led him to fight with peers and to 'lose it' in the playground.*
- Children with low self-esteem: for example, *Shona is a big girl for her age. Her pretty older sister is in the class above; comparisons are always being made and Shona has no sense of self-worth.*
- Children who have difficult relationships with their mother and miss their father: for example, *Shelley is very critical of herself and others. She cannot tolerate being shown where she can improve her work and interprets helpful attempts from peers and staff as criticism. She continually puts herself down. She fears taking risks and learning new tasks.*
- Children who are suffering from bereavement: for example, *Jamila's little brother was killed in a car accident. Jamila's mum and family are so overcome with grief that they have forgotten that Jamila also needs to mourn.*

Rationale for group work

Dramatherapists, because of our training, are ideally suited to run therapeutic groups in school. We all live and work in small or large groups; the human condition is inherently social, so therapeutic work in schools in a group setting is of equal validity with individual one-to-one work. Furthermore, children in schools are familiar with working in small learning groups.

Sylvia McNamara and Gill Moreton (2001) suggest that sometimes teachers avoid putting pupils with emotional and behavioural difficulties into situations that they (the teachers) judge the children might find difficult. And this applies to group work; some teachers believe that these children need one-to-one work only. This may lead to the isolation of the children with social, emotional and behavioural difficulties, and it leaves them with no positive opportunity to practise social skills themselves and to witness the modelling of good social skills by their peers.

Where there are limited resources in terms of time and money, group work is cost effective and short-term groups in schools over a term have been found to have effective outcomes. However, the selection of group members is crucial to the successful running of groups. The project coordinator might feel inclined to group together a number of children whose behaviour is causing them grief. However, I suggest that it is unwise to have, say, a group of six boys referred for acting out and aggression working together in a therapeutic group. Nor, in my view, is it appropriate to have six shy girls working together. Good practice indicates that a mixture of children referred with *moderate* levels of emotional behavioural and social difficulties, with as much of a mix of referral reasons, gender and ethnicity as possible, is the most effective for group formation.

The referral process

- *Leaflet*: First of all, it is important that parents are informed of the provision the school is making to give emotional support to children. I suggest that a leaflet explaining the project is sent out to all the parents to tell them about the intervention, its aims and which staff are involved.
- *Identification of children*: The project coordinator is responsible for identifying the children for emotional support and who will talk to the parents and tell them about the service and get their written permission for the dramatherapist to work with their child.
- *Referral form*: The dramatherapist makes an appointment to meet the child's teacher and to fill in a referral form. This form monitors the work. It is really important that the therapist and the teacher work together to discuss the child and then for them to speak again after the contract is over. (A suggested referral form is given in appendix A.) Because there is a pre-intervention measure and a post-intervention measure, there is a way of quantifying change; the perceptions of change are qualitative measures.
- *Parental consent*: it is the responsibility of the coordinator to make sure that they see the written parental consent before one-to-one work starts with children in primary school. However, it is equally the responsibility of the dramatherapist to check that the parent has given permission. Personally, I think it is advisable to meet the parent and to talk about the child and also to explain what dramatherapy involves. It is also essential to gain consent from the child.
- *Documents*: there should be a lockable cabinet for the files on each child; the suggestion is that it should be in the responsibility of the coordinator of the project.

The therapeutic contract with the child or the group of children

In my view, work with children in school should be contained within a period of a term with the opportunity to review; work with a particular child should be contained within the school year for developmental reasons. My experience tells me that small group work should be contained within a term. We can always review the work, make an ending, have a pause and then, if it is appropriate, make a new contract.

It is, of course, essential for the dramatherapist to make a contract with each child and each small group, allowing the children to say what they would like to be included and also to discuss the limitations of confidentiality and the safeguarding issues. Therefore the dramatherapist would present a contract of six to eight sessions with the possibility of a review, based on discussions on progress with the school project coordinator. Children will have the experience of making an anticipated ending with their therapist, which is something they may not have experienced before. Schools, in my experience, are notoriously bad at making endings (Greenhalgh 1994)!

Working with the children

Depending upon the age of the child, it is usual to set aside a whole hour for one-to-one work. If the child is very young and in reception class, you may think it appropriate to allocate 45 minutes. Group work is often the duration of a class period. In my experience as a dramatherapist and as a clinical supervisor, I think it is advisable, if not essential, to have co-workers, who could be a learning support staff member, to help keep the group safe. It is good practice to collect the child or children from class and take theme back to the class. My advice would be to make the contract between dramatherapist and child or children in the first session. Particularly important are the safeguarding issues, when we have the responsibility of explaining the limits of confidentiality.

It is also important, I suggest, to evaluate, where possible, the child's perception of dramatherapy and her relationship with the therapist. Appendix B contains a 'Children's evaluation form', which I have used successfully in school. Of course, some children will need help to understand what she or he is being asked to do. Some children might like to tell the therapist what to say and others might also like to draw a picture to illustrate.

The room and the resources

What is needed? There needs to be a private room or space where no one can overhear or interrupt. This is often hard to find in crowded schools, but in my view it is essential to keep the child and children *safe*, and for the work to be safe. An open space where people pass by and children can peer around screens is not suitable. Also, one needs sufficient space for dramatherapy, which is sometimes hard to negotiate.

There needs to be a viewing window at adult height in the door, which should never be locked during sessions for health and safety reasons.

Ideally, the room should have a sink or at least a bowl of water, with cloths for wiping up and tissues, paper towels, and pinnies for painting work. Children's files should be kept in a locked filing cabinet.

Resources should include sand trays: one for wet sand and one for dry sand; little people/small animals/shells etc. for working in the sand, and creative materials: coloured paper, pens, felt tips, clay, playdough, paints, brushes, fabric for dressing up, hats and model cars – including ambulances and police cars.

Conclusion

In this chapter, I have presented a model of the provision of emotional support in primary schools, which covers the setting up and management of the project. A possible referral form, which has qualitative and quantitative aspects, is included in appendix A. I have suggested that the training of registered dramatherapists and other arts therapists and play therapists, with its emphasis on working creatively through metaphor and symbol, makes them ideally placed to work with troubled children in school.

References

Bowlby, J. (1988) *A Secure Base: Clinical Applications of Attachment Theory*. London: Routledge.

Department for Education (2008) *Children and young people in mind: the final report of the National CAMHS Review*. London: HMSO.

Gerhardt, S. (2004) *Why Love Matters: How Affection Shapes a Baby's Brain*. London: Bruner Routledge.

Greenhalgh, P. (1994) *Emotional Growth and Learning*. London: Routledge.

Howe, D. (2005) *Child Abuse and Neglect: Attachment, Development & Intervention*. Palgrave Macmillan.

McNamara, S. and Moreton, G. (2001) *Managing Behaviour*. London: David Fulton.

Siegel, D.F. and Hartzell, M. (2003) *Parenting from the Inside Out*. New York: Tarcher Penguin.

Appendix A

Internal referral and evaluation form

Part 1: Referral

School... Date of referral: ....

Name of referrer/position: ....

Class teacher's name (if different): ....

Name of child... Date of birth.................

M/F Age........... Year group.................

Name of dramatherapist ....

Figure 1 Internal referral and evaluation form.

Part 2: Contract

The work may not proceed without the knowledge and agreement of the parent/carer and the child. Please indicate when you met the parent and when you met the child and confirm that agreement has been given.

The child: Date met…................. Agreement? Yes/no

The parent/carer: Date met.............. Agreement? Yes/no

Number of sessions............ Day of session:........... Time of session:.........

Start date: .... Planned end date:...........................

Any further comments about the referral:

Figure 2 Contract.

Part 3: Degree of concern

This part of the referral form should be filled in while you are having a discussion with the child's teacher/referrer before your contract with the child starts. You are asking the teacher to be specific about the reasons why she or he is referring the child for dramatherapy. What is it about the child's behaviour that causes the concern; for example, the teacher might want to refer a child because she seems to be 'depressed'. You will ask the teacher to be specific about the behaviours that make her think the child is 'depressed'. Then you write down three specific behaviours. (It may be that the child is often 'tearful', 'does not engage in the lesson', 'is often absent because she is sick'.) You then ask the teacher to rate her degree of concern.

Could you please tell me what three concerns you have about the child; please be specific. Please mark your degree of concern from 1 to 5, where 5 is high concern.

Before dramatherapy begins: Degree of concern

	1	2	3	4	5
1.					
2.					
3.					

What hopes do you have for the child after this dramatherapy contract is completed? *(Please be specific. For example, if you would like the child to be happier, say how would you know in behavioural terms if the child were happier.)*

Teacher's signature: Date:

Figure 3 Degree of concern form.

The dramatherapist goes to see the teacher after the contract with the child is over in order to see if the teacher sees any change in the child.

Teacher's name: Date:

Please indicate where the child is now in relation to the concerns you had at the beginning.

After dramatherapy ends: Degree of concern

	1	2	3	4	5
1.					
2.					
3.					

Were your hopes for this work fulfilled?
(please be specific in behavioural terms)

Completely/partially/not at all

Other comments:

Dramatherapist's comments:

Figure 4 When the contract is over.

Appendix B

After dramatherapy/Children's evaluation form

Dramatherapist: Date:

Child/young person:

Before you came to see me, how were you feeling?

☹☹ ☹ 😐 ☺ ☺☺

How are you feeling now?

☺☺ ☺ 😐 ☹ ☹☹

What was good about coming to see me?

I wonder what was hard or difficult?

Who should come to dramatherapy, do you think?

Thank you very much for answering my questions.

Signed:

Figure 5 Post-intervention Children's evaluation form.

24 Holding the family in the heart of school

Lauraine Leigh

Introduction

This book concerns a range of models and in this chapter the focus is on what I refer to as the Dovetail model of dramatherapy, drawn from Jennings' EPR developmental model of dramatherapy (1990). The Dovetail model appears to provide a framework for attachment and separation issues in the furtherance of enabling the child's wellbeing and desire for learning.

This chapter includes a discussion of the difficulties in engaging parents. A vignette linking theory and practice then illustrates family dramatherapy with a 13-year-old boy diagnosed with Attention Deficit Hyperactivity Disorder (ADHD) and Oppositional Defiant Disorder (ODD). The boy lived with his single parent and siblings in a White UK family. The child's teachers were concerned about his challenging, violent behaviour in class, and his lack of interest in learning. An amalgam method, which ensures case integrity and confidentiality, draws on families from different cultures and ethnicities. The chapter concludes with reference to evaluations from teachers, parents and young people.

Jennings' EPR model and the Dovetail model

The Dovetail model is based on Jennings' developmental model of dramatherapy (1990) which has three stages: embodiment, projection and role (EPR). The Dovetail model works for me in schools because it makes use of psychoanalytic concepts that seem to parallel and add another dimension to Jennings' model.

As stated, the aim of the Dovetail model is to provide a framework for attachment and separation issues in the furtherance of enabling the child's wellbeing and desire for learning. It is informed by several theories, including Winnicott's transitional object (Winnicott 2003 [1958]: 233), Bowlby's work on attachment (Bowlby 1988), Klein's work on splitting psychopathology and the depressive position (Klein 1998 [1975]: 199), and Bion's work on containment (Symington and Symington 1999: 50–58).

Embodiment means literally working with a focus on the body, working with the senses and a variety of materials, for instance a sponge football, flowers, soft dough. This includes action, physicality, touch, sound, scents. As Dix (chapter 5) points out, the developmental continuum EPR can be worked through sequentially and returned to as necessary.

Projection is a term used in both dramatherapy and psychoanalysis, with different although linked meanings. 'Projection of aspects of oneself is preceded by Denial: i.e. one denies that one feels such and such an emotion . . . but asserts that someone else does' (Rycroft 1972). Through dramatherapy's safe distancing using story and metaphor, inner worlds can be made safe enough to reflect on. There is a clear difference in the use of the term *Projection* in the EPR model in dramatherapy. Here 'projection' in the developmental model refers to the child or client projecting aspects of the self into an object or an artefact. A little girl with Asperger's disorder might animate a puppet to jump about. The dramatherapist or psychotherapist would generally feel that the puppet represents the child's projection of her own lively feelings, possibly as they relate to being with the therapist. 'Dramatherapy emphasises the ways in which projection can be linked to dramatic form to enable a client to create, discover and engage with external representations of inner conflicts' (Jones 2007: 140).

To work towards the third stage in the linear development in EPR, *Role*, the therapist might work a second puppet alongside the child, beginning to develop a puppet story. The child might then be able to get into a role, using her own body perhaps to impersonate the puppet character (Jones 1996: 107). US dramatherapist Renee Emunah, working with young people and universality, writes that dramatic play in therapy 'results in a process that is most often pleasurable' (Emunah 1994: 5). In the vignette we look at a familiar scene 'in any classroom in the world' using a similar dynamic.

Conscious that working with EPR combined with aspects of psychoanalytic thinking involves working towards maturity, I go into a session wondering whether the young client can begin the process of maturation, beginning with embodiment and then projection. Will they be able to work with role-play? Autistic children for instance are often unable to 'put themselves into someone else's shoes', but I agree with Tytherleigh and Karkou (2010: 213) that autistic children can fleetingly take on a role. For instance, I have observed a child 'feeding a doll as if it is a baby'. The ability to symbolize is the beginning of a small but significant move along the spectrum away from concrete, rigid thinking (Segal 2000 [1991]: 33). So the question arises: does the ability to begin to get into a role, to work with role-play and role-reversal, enable a move onwards towards maturity?

Engaging families: family dramatherapy and multi-disciplinary working

Initiatives to work with the whole family, where possible, have been a focus since Every Child Matters (Department for Education and Skills 2003) and The Common Assessment Framework. Governments change. Continuity and offering family dramatherapy helps the child fundamentally. By offering a psychoanalytically based model in schools, we are also offering help for parents who themselves often need emotional support. Rustin points out they may be offered a Parent Partnership model when they would actually like to be able to express their own needs and have them worked with. 'The unconscious is being ruled out as a significant factor once partnership is interpreted in a way which is designed to avoid recognising dependence on the therapist, and to assert equality, when the reality is that one person needs something that the other may be able to help them find' (Rustin 2009: 208).

As Roger has identified with such clarity (chapter 13), dramatherapists need to create and maintain constant ongoing communication with teachers, headteachers and management for all aspects of therapy in educational settings. The use of a boundaried therapeutic space in schools also has good implications, for teacher–parent relationships as well as for the child and parent at home. Therapeutic space in schools signifies more than physical space. Being together in a quiet space, without interruption and with the time to think together, is bedrock for the work. Family dramatherapy organically develops a mediation role, and sometimes there is an anger management focus. The dramatherapist must establish and keep the therapeutic space and maintain its boundaries so that people can say difficult things to each other. Working with all members of the family creates the opportunity not only for discussion, but most usefully when words can run out, for just *being together*: for non-verbal intervention.

Therapeutic containment and boundaries

Boundaries (chapter 1) are complementary to school rules, and it is essential to agree them with all concerned before sessions can begin. Agreeing a boundary does not of course mean that it will not be challenged within family work. Where in classrooms teachers use school rules and discipline in order to be able to teach the class, differently – and in a complementary way – in the school therapy room, the therapeutic space and boundaries enable the dramatherapist and family to think about what is happening if the boundaries are pushed or broken. Family and therapist can look curiously together at why that may be happening. Envy can sometimes play a component part. This can sometimes helpfully be represented within dramatic form, and sometimes directly addressed together.

Referrals and assessment

As Haythorne (chapter 18) identifies, referrals come from concerned parents, as well as any member of the multi-disciplinary team. Young people may refer themselves initially through a 'drop in' session. Information is appropriately shared by the multi-disciplinary team through the

Common Assessment Framework (CAF). For family work it is important for the family to be able to tell their story to the dramatherapist. Questions are part of our work for assessments, but they can be difficult and painful for parents and children where there are pressing emotional difficulties and needs. We need to be sensitive with parents, who can themselves be vulnerable. The way we ask what we ask, and the way we think about things together with the family is important. Family dramatherapy aims to enable schools to help and to keep chaotic, troubled children, rather in the spirit of Davies and Burdett's New Zealand Families and Schools Together (FAST) *Creating the conditions for saner societies* (2004: 277).

Encouragement and the concept of being good enough

Geddes (2006: 120) writes of the importance of positive encouragement for children's brain development. Looking wider, the question arises: could our education system be helped to think differently about the term 'excellence'? Andrew Samuels (2000) focused on Winnicott's term 'good enough', asking what happens if we say we have a good enough education system. He suggested an attitude of tolerance enables us to avoid the 'inevitable paralysis that follows on massive disappointment'. In a similar vein, Klein warned of the 'psychological difficulties and striking personality changes' for children around puberty, pointing out that teachers and parents can feel unequal to the considerable needs children have at this time. Many parents will 'spur their child on when what he needs is holding back, or else fail to give encouragement when he wants their confidence and trust' (Klein 1991: 54).

Children and young people crossing wide demographics live in single parent families, which can present a stressful environment. At times these children and parents feel vulnerable, keenly aware of separation and loss, which can stir up difficult feelings of abandonment, grief, anger and envy. Parent and child can develop an intense, enmeshed or 'entangled' relationship (Fonagy et al. 1993: 964) relationship where a parent relates to their young child as if the child is parenting them, or the substitute for the other parent, as if the child can think and feel as the adult does. Young (2001: 3) writes accessibly about the Oedipal triangle, 'intermingled and as lifelong unconscious preoccupations which have ramifications throughout both personal and large-scale history'. In a nutshell, these primitive, earliest feelings refer to a desire to possess the parent of the opposite sex and eliminate that of the same sex. If not resolved, these feelings can continue and cause problems with maturity (Rycroft 1972: 105). In such cases it is possible to observe a child and parent each feel a sense of confusion, an inability to either think or speak for themselves. This affects the child's learning process.

In this section of the book (V) we look at future potential for dramatherapy in schools. Fonagy and Bateman (2006: 84) helpfully focus on 'normal' relationships, the core self; 'a sense of constancy'. Childhood is about developing one's core self: a delicate mental health process. How does this sit in schools today? As Haigh points out (chapter 25), schools are implicated in this mental process. As a dramatherapist, I have often seen dramatherapy help change patterns of Winnicott's 'paralysis', or low self-esteem in children, and with families and schools. We are working preventatively, frequently with difficult attachment patterns and separations, where sometimes there have been negative intergenerational family patterns (Fraiberg et al. 1980).

A further aspect of today's shifts in culture is the transition experienced when a new step-parent comes into the family. Many families manage this change well; however, it can feel challenging to some children, who now share their parent with a comparative stranger. Feelings of closeness to the parent, of feeling excluded and 'not being good enough', can be around for these children, compounding oedipal difficulties around 'reaching the depressive position', around reaching maturity.

How psychoanalytic thinking adds depth

At the Second European Conference of Child and Adolescent Mental Health in Educational Settings, Naples 2007, the programme read:

> The importance that education plays in the development of children and adolescents, and children's experience of failure is widely accepted as having an impact upon the mental health of young people and their families.

Conference keynote speaker Mireille Cifali Bega, psychoanalyst and Professor of Education in Geneva said: 'Psychoanalysis enables us to go on thinking whenever some form of resistance emerges' and she suggested Freud's views on education need to be constantly interpreted and reinterpreted because education is a world where 'judgemental attitudes and opprobrium are almost inevitably present' (2007; Official programme translation). In schools we are working very much with the super-ego (Sandler, Holder, Dare and Dreher 2005 [1997]: 27), a force that can persecute, or do the opposite, enliven.

We can all identify with the kind of uncomfortable, even overwhelming feeling that going into a school stirs up. Many parents may have painful memories of their own difficult schooling. Feelings can include an inner sense of shame or anxiety, which are often displaced as anger towards teachers. A fundamental aspect of family work is to engage reluctant, anxious parents from the widest backgrounds and cultures, but official stationery sent to parents can be off-putting (Standing 1998). Therapists' work needs to 'contain' (Bion 1984 [1963]: 6) difficult feelings, and differences – just as mothers and fathers, together or divided, do well to continue to communicate so as to contain, to hold, their child's feelings (Waddell 2005). A psychotherapy room within school symbolizes containment for difficult feelings in schools. 'Schools show variable capacities to function as effective "containers" of both feelings and attributes that can otherwise be disowned, split off and projected into others' (Music 2007).

Separation and attachment issues

Contacting and finally meeting the family in school can take a great deal of work. We need to work with parent and child with an acknowledgement of difficulties and anxieties – and hopes – they may have. The aim is to enable more effective communication, even a warmer relationship between those who live together, whilst also enabling each family member to feel more a sense of their own personal boundaries. In clarifying this, the therapist, working psychodynamically with the family, is enabling the child to feel more aware of his or her likes and dislikes, to feel more listened to by mum or dad or step parents. The aim is that we all work towards enabling the child to feel stronger. If the child's resilience is strengthened *with the parent present* he will be more likely to be curious about learning in class and more able to speak appropriately with his peers and with his teachers. Winnicott stated that in working with the parent in the service of the child, we are actually helping the parent themselves (Winnicott 2003 [1958]: 308). It is possible 'to take the child's side against the parent and *at the same time* to gain and keep the parents' confidence' (2003 [1956]: 93). Bowlby's ethological approach to attachment issues highlights the need of the child for an emotionally warm and secure relationship. 'It is just as necessary for analysts to study the way a child is really treated as it is to study the internal representations he has . . . the principal focus of our studies should be the interaction of the one with the other' (Bowlby 2010 [1988]: 49). Psychodynamically the therapist looks at how we are relating to each other in the session, how that feels, and we think about the possible meanings of it. There are times when interpretation is useful; equally there are times when it is not.

Pleasure in learning

Anna Freud identified inhibitions to learning as equating with not being able to work through the Oedipus complex, and she urged that educationalists and parents should be enlightened about this work (Sandler 1992: 103). In 1930, Klein identified the epistomophilic instinct (1998 [1975]: 227), linking the ability to symbolize with learning. She enabled her clients to reach what she identified as the 'depressive position' (Klein 1998 [1975]: 344–369). Where strong feelings and inhibitions are concerned, she wrote:

> the results of even years of pedagogical labour present no relation to the effort expended, while in analysis we often find these inhibitions removed in a comparatively short time and replaced by complete pleasure in learning. (1998 [1975]: 54)

Families and struggling

Family dramatherapy in schools appears to enable a developmental move forward for the child. There appears to be a parallel that aligns Jennings' EPR developmental process with Klein's two psychoanalytical positions, which Bion termed mathematically PS – D (Symington and Symington 1999: 94). Bion's work on this model links with my observations when working through EPR.

We are not framing ideas with a cognitive ethos. We are working to acknowledge inner worlds, difficult feelings. This can feel a struggle. Families can put all their difficult feelings onto the therapist, who needs to be robust, to contain the emotions, to interpret with great sensitivity (Music 2007: 17).

Jason's vignette

Background

Jason, 13, was halfway through Year 8 and had been diagnosed with Attention Deficit Hyperactivity Disorder (ADHD) during primary school. Both at school and at home, he could not sit still. He roved around and called out inappropriately, demanding constant attention from either the teacher or his mother. Heated challenges, arguments and fights were his way of communicating. He had now been diagnosed with ODD, oppositional defiant disorder, 'a recurrent pattern of negativitistic, defiant, disobedient and hostile behaviour towards authority figures that persists for at least 6 months' (DSM-IV-TR 2000). However, his sports teacher praised his football skills. Jason's school was on the verge of considering his exclusion. His psychiatrist had prescribed ritalin, but his mother was not keen. It is at these times that dramatherapy, neither a reward nor a punishment, can help in schools.

Assessment meeting

At the first dramatherapy meeting, the boundaries immediately help parent and child feel supported. Parent and child understand they speak for themselves, and do not have to speak. At this initial assessment meeting with the parent only, there is a focus on how the parent sees their child's difficulty, the child's parentage and important separations and losses, and siblings – because 'everyone fears to be dethroned in childhood. . . – a core experience of playmates and peers' (Mitchell 2003: 2). The child's infancy, eating and sleeping habits hold an important key. Details of the separated birth parent are important (does the child see them?) and whether grandparents/family live nearby or help. When I then meet the young person with their parent, I ask them for their own idea of their ability in Maths and English, and whether they think there is 'anything ok about English, Maths and school?' The aim is thus to include the learning process in a core way and from the child's point of view, within a useful holistic overview of their emotional difficulties.

Jason's father had left the family home three years earlier. The mother, Jason and his two sisters aged four and eight, lived near the maternal grandparents. Mum had nothing positive to say about separated dad, who lived two hours away. I later felt the boy's vulnerability and pain as he cringed at his mother's disparaging tone towards dad, who Jason saw on birthdays and at Christmas. Dad and his new partner had a new baby. The mother confided the information before Jason joined us that Jason had once taken money from her purse (Winnicott 2003 [1958]: 309).

Jason was tall and looked older than 13. He was brought by the SENCO towards the end of the meeting, so the four of us could think together about whether family dramatherapy might be helpful for him, and whether he felt he could keep the boundaries of the work. Jason looked uncomfortable to be with three adults. I acknowledged his and his mother's courage in being there. He agreed with the SENCO and his mother that he would like some help and thought he would like to try to keep the boundaries.

The first session

Jason was reluctant to come in with his mother, beginning a conversation with another pupil outside the room. When he did come in, I decided to address this avoidance by wondering aloud and mildly if he thought I was not able to be of any use to him. I also offered a boundary, a length of wool once helpful in a school where a famous footballer had been a pupil a few years before. Jason became calmer and more focused and began to look more at me and mum as he spoke.

We thought about the boundaries for the sessions: 'No put-downs' and 'You can say "Pass"'. I explained these, and invited Jason and his mother to stand somewhere on the wool line. At one end this would mean: 'I'm fairly sure I can keep the boundaries', and at the other: 'I don't feel strong about keeping the boundaries so I might need some help'. Jason stood at the 'fairly sure' positive end, mum actually stood behind him. Jason might not control his anger in class, but he stood at the positive end. This indicated his hopes, which I remarked on.

Not unexpectedly, Jason continually pushed the boundaries over six sessions. From the assessment, my own observations of his engagement with the sessions and my knowledge of his situation, my feeling was there were likely to be feelings of exclusion and jealousy for Jason. Mum tended to idealize her daughter and be rather indulgent about Jason's unruly temper. This is not uncommon with mums and sons.

Jason now threw a softball at the wall and caught it every time. I complimented him on his skills, and asked if we might join in. He stopped, as if disciplined. I reminded Jason that in these sessions he had choices and no obligation to join in. Would Jason like to work with some colour? He looked at the array of paints and glanced at mum, who looked interested, and he thought he would. The mother looked at me hopefully and joined him quietly at the table, where they settled next to each other, mum keen to choose her colours from several tubes of acrylic. Jason chose his colours less certainly. Mum began using swirling movements on a sheet of paper. Jason asked her if she would draw the same on his paper. My work needed to be sensitive and tentative: it was important they should not feel or be hurried or interrupted, that they should feel 'held' particularly at the start of the containment process. Segal links the later capacity for symbolisation and thinking with 'a good relationship between container and contained' (1989: 5).

Embodiment, touch and finding words

Parent and child can begin to feel a sense of acceptance in therapy. As they sat close together I was reminded of the effect of non-intrusive touch, known to be life-affirming: 'without physical touch, the baby cannot flourish' (Orbach 2004: 40).

In 'Before the threshold: destruction, reparation and creativity in relation to the depressive position', Judith Edwards (2005), working with developmental issues, suggests the threshold of creativity may be a transitional development before the depressive position is reached. I think this applies here. Describing the dread and hope around this, Edwards links it to 'a fundamental human endeavour not solely to do with guilt and the desire to repair, but also with an innate drive to participate in human discourse' (2005: 318).

Recapping: Jason is in a chaotic state in the classroom (though not in sports lessons). Here, while they painted together, mum and son began making cooing sounds. They were absorbed for some time, leaning against each other in their own world. I sat observing them together, their choice of colours and their movements and shapes, their different pressure on the brushes and felt tips, their hesitation and pleasure in making colour choices, their process of painting. Jason and his mum painted the spaces in between the swirls on their own paper. Both were as if in a hand and upper body dance using aspects of movement, sight and touch, sniffing the paint, sitting side by side, expressing themselves colourfully, carefully on paper. I was conscious of these endearing musical sounds. Witnessing one another, being witnessed by me, suggested a contribution towards 'self-coherence', each one to a sense of a core self (Stern 2000: 71).

The Oedipal context

The mother had mentioned to me privately that 18 months earlier she and dad had tried to get back together again, and that Jason had got into her bed at the weekends when she and Jason's father got up. I wondered about Jason's oedipal issues now – mum and Jason, mum and new boyfriend; Jason's father whom he hardly saw, who now had a new baby and family.

Finishing his painting, Jason sat back, watching mum, waiting for her to finish painting. His complete absorption in this process reminded me of a baby who has had a good feed and who sits back from the breast, satisfied, calm. At this point the grandfather's voice was heard outside. He had arrived early to collect them. Even though Jason indicated by a quick shared look at mum that he could hear his grandfather's voice, this young man diagnosed with ADHD and ODD was quiet, 'contained'. With mum still painting, he remained focused, watching her painting, waiting calmly.

We all looked at their paintings. They were interested in how different they were, and how similar. Finally in a circle, each of us in turn made a bodily 'freeze frame', adding a sound, expressing physically how the session had felt. These were 'mirrored' back by us. Jason quickly shrugged then stretched upwards, adding, 'ok'. Mum clapped. If Jason had a sudden self-consciousness about clapping back to mum, he nevertheless joined in.

It seemed this work enabled for both Jason and Mum a feeling of balance, even of comfortable fullness, a feeling of curiosity and of more tolerance and resilience.

Later stages

A week later Jason worked with the 'As If' game. He chose a card to mime with gesture, body shape and movement, wanting us to guess his mime. 'Scoring a winning goal' opened up the subject of when he is praised at school for football skills. Mum described feeling proud, which pleased Jason. 'You feel special to mum', I said. I talked gently about how we can also feel sibling jealousy, when siblings seem perfect. He made eye contact with his mother and she thought about how she feels different with each of her children. Was she ever jealous of her siblings? She was. After Jason expressed some envy of his sisters, mother and son thought about how they both might find some special time weekly at home to chat and paint, just the two of them. Jason was able to think about whether a boy who is good at sport and team games could possibly also sit companionably with classmates in Maths.

In the penultimate session Jason role played 'a boy who comes late into the classroom. The only seat left in the classroom is next to the dreaded classroom bully'. This two-chair model (L. Leigh 2002, personal communication) holds a useful key for working with resilience. Jason immediately expressed violence towards 'the dreaded classroom bully': 'I'd smash him'.

We were able to remind ourselves of the boundaries, and also think about how this boy might just feel the need to 'lord it' over others. Jason began to reflect and even try out different ways of being with this kind of boy, which might also help him, Jason. I praised Jason for keeping the boundaries of the session.

Strengthening a young person's resilience involves helping him feel he can approach difficult things. Classrooms are full of rivalrous feelings, along with feelings of failure and inadequacy. Here we worked with Jason's ego, through the use of role and role reversal. His own feelings were projected in role into finally sitting as 'the late boy in any classroom in the world who has to sit next to "the class bully"'. Lousada refers to the pressing cultural relevance of 'the *we* ego . . . which can be learnt through sibling/peer encounters . . . (which have) social and political implications, especially . . . in view of youth knife crime' (2009: 23). Here, we wondered, could Jason prepare this scene by standing behind the bully's chair, suggesting the words this 'classroom bully' might say to this 'late boy'? He was able to create a dialogue between the two boys, working with his own projections each time, sitting to role-play. His mother chose to watch from the witnessing space. The ability to work with role-reversal enables the young person to begin to feel stronger, to see a situation from a distance. The therapist sometimes 'sits in' for the characters.

This work is essentially integrative. De-roleing ensures child and therapist are not left identified with either 'bully' or 'victim'. Jason's mother was surprised he had been able to put himself into the shoes of the sort of boy he feared. She said she and her sister had been bullied at school, news for Jason. It was helpful to think a little about this together. In the final evaluation session we thought about how each of us can sometimes act in bullying ways, and how we can sometimes realize we are being bullied.

Conclusion

Evaluations show children feel stronger about being in class with peers and teacher. They like being listened to by their family, miming 'As If', painting, creating scenes with their family, trying out different ways of being and behaving, being witnessed by their family. They report feeling more able to ask for help in class.

I praised Jason for keeping the boundaries of the session (chapter 1). Parents report less family stress, increased tolerance, feeling more inclined to listen and talk with their children and step-children.

Teachers' evaluations (see chapter 1, figure 1) have shown significant improvements in young people's ability to listen, cooperate and communicate with their peers; speaking skills in class are often more appropriate. This suggests the child has more *desire* to learn.

Family dramatherapy appears to address core family issues and enable integrative links between creativity, communication, emotional support and learning. The methodology of the Dovetail model, which links Jennings' EPR developmental model of dramatherapy with psychoanalytic concepts, is more detailed than described. Further research is needed.

References

Bion, W. R. (1962) *Learning from Experience*. London: Heinemann; repr. Maresfield Reprints, London: Karnac.

Bion, W. R. (1984 [1963]) *Elements of Psycho-Analysis*. London: Karnac Books.

Bowlby, J. (2010 [1988]) *A Secure Base: Clinical Applications of Attachment Theory. Psychoanalysis as Art and Science*. London: Routledge.

Cifali Bega, Mereille (2007) Relationships in schools: contemporary problems and opportunities. Keynote address, Second European Conference on Child and Adolescent Mental Health in Educational Settings, Naples. Official translation.

Davies, E. and Burdett, J. (2004) 'Creating the conditions for saner societies', in Read, J., Mosher, L. R., and Bentall, R. P. (eds.), *Models of Madness: Psychological, Social and Biological Approaches to Schizophrenia*. The International Society for the Psychological Treatments of the Schizophrenias and Other Psychoses. Hove: Brunner Routledge.

Department for Education and Skills (2003) *Every Child Matters*. London: The Stationery Office.

DSM-IV-TR (2000) *Diagnostic and Statistical Manual of Mental Disorders, Fourth Edition Text Revision*. Washington, DC: American Psychiatric Association.

Edwards, J. (2005) 'Before the threshold: destruction, reparation and creativity in relation to the depressive position'. *Journal of Child Psychotherapy*, 31 (3), 317–334.

Emunah, R. (1994) *Acting for Real*. London: Psychology Press.

Fonagy, P. and Bateman, A. (2006) *Mentalisation-Based Treatment for Borderline Personality Disorder: A Practical Guide*. Oxford: Oxford University Press.

Fonagy, P., Steele, M., Moran, G., Steele, H., and Higgitt, A. (1993) 'Measuring the Ghost in the Nursery: An empirical study of the relation between parents' mental representations of childhood experiences and their infants' security of attachment'. *Journal of the American Psychoanalytic Association*, 41, 957–989.

Fraiberg, S., Adelson, E., and Shapiro, V. (1980) *Ghosts in the Nursery: A psychoanalytical Approach to the Problems of Impaired Infant–Mother Relationships*. London: Tavistock.

Geddes, H. (2006) *Attachment in the Classroom*. Bath: Worth Publishing.

Jennings, S. (1990) *Dramatherapy with Families, Groups and Individuals*. London: Jessica Kingsley.

Jones, P. (1996) *Drama as Therapy, Theatre as Living*. London: Routledge.

Jones, P. (2007) *Drama as Therapy: Theory, Practice and Research*. London: Routledge.

Klein, M. (1991) 'Inhibitions and difficulties at puberty' [1922], in *Love, Guilt and Reparation*, 54–58. London: Virago.

Klein, M. (1998 [1975]) *Love, Guilt and Reparation and Other Works 1921–1945*. London: Vintage.

—— Inhibitions and Difficulties at Puberty (1922): 54–58.

—— Personification in the Play of Children (1929): 199.

—— The Importance of Symbol-Formation in the Development of the Ego (1930): 75.

—— The Oedipus Complex in the light of early anxieties (1945): 370–419.

Lousada, O. (2009) *Hidden Twins. What Adult Opposite Sex Twins Have To Teach Us*. London: Karnac.

Mitchell, J. (2003) *Siblings: Sex and Violence*. Cambridge: Polity.

Music, G. (2007) 'Learning Our Lessons: Some issues arising from delivering mental health services in school settings'. *Journal of Psychoanalytic Psychotherapy* 21 (1), 1–19.

Orbach, S. (2004) 'The body in clinical practice. Part One. There is no such thing as a body', in White, K. (ed.), *Touch: Attachment and the Body*, 17–34. London: Karnac.

Rustin, M. (2009) 'Work with parents', in Lanyado, M. and Horne, A. (eds.), *The Handbook of Child & Adolescent Psychotherapy: Psychoanalytic Approaches*, 206–219. London: Routledge.

Rycroft, C. A. (1972) *A Critical Dictionary of Psychoanalysis*. London: Penguin Books.

Samuels, A. (2000) Presentation to Psychotherapists and Counsellors for Social Responsibility Conference. *Psychotherapy and the Political Domain – Politics on the Couch: Citizenship and the Internal Life*. (Private record).

Sandler, J. (1992) *Anna Freud: The Harvard Lectures*. London: Karnac and The Institute of Psychoanalysis.

Sandler, J., Holder, A., Dare, C., and Dreher, C. U. (2005 [1997]) *Freud's Models of the Mind*. London: Karnac.

Segal, H. (1989) 'Introduction', in Britton, R., Feldman, M., and O'Shaughnessy, E. (eds.), *The Oedipus Complex Today Clinical Implications*. London: Karnac.

Segal, H. (2000 [1991]) *Dream, Phantasy and Art*. The New Library of Psychoanalysis Vol. 12, Spillius, E. B. (Ed.). London: Routledge and the Institute of Psychoanalysis.

Standing, K. (1998) 'Writing the voices of the less powerful – research on lone mothers', in Edwards, R. and Ribbens, J. (eds.), *Feminist Dilemmas in Qualitative Research: Public Knowledge and Private Lives*. London: Sage.

Stern, D. N. (2000) *The Interpersonal World of the Infant. A View from Psychoanalysis and Developmental Psychology*. London: Basic Books.

Symington, J. and Symington, N. (1999) *The Clinical Thinking of Wilfred Bion*. London: Routledge.

Tytherley, L. and Karkou, V. (2010) 'Dramatherapy, autism and relationship building: a case study', in Karkou, V. (ed.), *Arts Therapies in Schools: Research and Practice*. London: Jessica Kingsley.

Waddell M. (2005) Lecture, *Adolescence: A Narcissistic Disorder*. Institute of Psychoanalysis.

Winnicott, D. W. (2003 [1958]) *Through Paediatrics to Psychoanalysis Collected Papers*. London: Karnac.

—— Reparation in Respect of Mother's Organized Defence against Depression (1948): 93.

—— The Antisocial Tendency (1956): 308.

Young, R. M. (2001) *The Oedipus Complex*. Ideas in Psychoanalysis. Cambridge: Icon Books.

25 Future possibilities

Rex Haigh

> Recent figures demonstrate that up to 10% of children and 20% of adolescents suffer from emotional and conduct disorders, a further 7–10% suffer from moderate to severe mental illness like anorexia and depression and suicide rates for boys aged 15–19 years are still on the increase. As many as 84,000 children and young people take anti-depressants, 480,000 children and young people aged from 5–15 years in the UK have clinically significant depression or anxiety.
>
> (Department of Health 2005)

This chapter is in the form of questions and answers, with questions put by Lauraine Leigh to Dr Rex Haigh, a consultant psychiatrist, clinical advisor to the National Personality Disorder Development Programme and training lead for the new National Personality Disorder Institute at Nottingham University. He is founder and project lead of the 'Community of Communities' quality network at the Royal College of Psychiatrists and is involved with several third-sector organizations, including the Association of Therapeutic Communities, Borderline UK, Personality Plus, Community Housing and Therapy, the Society for Psychotherapy Research and the British and Irish Group for the Study of Personality Disorder. Rex has written and published numerous articles about therapeutic communities and personality disorder, and is co-editor of both the Jessica Kingsley 'Community, Culture and Change' book series and the *International Journal of Therapeutic Communities*.

LL: Thank you for being included in this book, Rex. Having heard your talk to Reading Therapies Group several years ago about personality disorder, I made a connection with young people and school exclusion. A fundamental connection between schools and improved mental health in society is our book's focus and I know you are keen for an emphasis by the government on preventive ways of working with mental health issues in schools.

RH: Yes, the future potential of all members of society is largely determined by their 'primary emotional development' in childhood, through families, social networks and education. How much better it would be if this time of life could become the main focus of the government's 'public mental health' work, rather than picking up all the pieces in an over-stretched mental health system, or in a predominantly public-safety-orientated criminal justice system.

Emotional development is at the heart of everybody's adult personality: when it is disrupted and goes wrong, the consequences for the individual, their family and society at large are truly devastating. The 'National Personality Disorder Programme', funded by the Department of Health, Ministry of Justice and Department for Education, sees the challenge over a person's lifecourse.

LL: Your contribution here links children's lives with adult lives, and with emotional wellbeing. Schools are in a prime position to provide effective and appropriate mental health care and prevention.

We should perhaps look at the kinds of things that can go wrong for us as we develop into adults. In your position as a leading consultant psychiatrist, clinical advisor to the National Personality Disorder Development Programme, and training lead for the new National Personality Disorder Institute at Nottingham University, you have worked tirelessly to erase the term 'Personality Disorder'. As a group analyst, you refer to Foulkes' emphasis on the group, in a way – I'm paraphrasing – there's 'no such thing' as an individual (Foulkes 1990).

It is very useful to understand from you how you see dramatherapy and drama teaching fitting into children's emotional wellbeing. How and whether children in schools can be enabled to express their difficult and also hopeful feelings enough through the intervention of dramatherapy and the other arts therapies and play therapy within schools is a question at the heart of this book.

Connections between children's schooling and emotional wellbeing are highlighted in 'Part IV Evidence and outcomes'. 'Part II Case studies' shows the reader how dramatherapy helps children, groups and families to express difficult, painful feelings safely in schools.

Drama methods with children in schools as preventive measures

RH: In the days of pre-recession abundance and optimism, ideas abounded for further developments, including using drama methods with children in schools as a public mental health preventive measure.

LL: In this book we look at ways of increasing dramatherapy and emotional support in schools in several ways, for instance, in chapter 3, a dramatherapist and educational psychologist look at combining professional work in order to meet children's needs more widely.

RH: Although there seems to be little appetite in government for starting any large new initiatives at the moment, there may be a barely discernable groundswell of changing opinion, which is looking at different frameworks: 'small is beautiful', 'green care' and 'arts for health'.

LL: It is encouraging to link green, environmental issues with psychotherapeutic interventions, and your initiative 'Green Care' is a valuable, far-sighted initiative, opening doors for holistic ways of being with each other that do not harm, that acknowledge difference and choices, that are sustainable and life enhancing.

Specifically, schoolchildren learn about the environment from infant classes, therefore not surprisingly they have anxieties about the future. EcoPsychologists, Hilary Prentice (2003) and Mary-Jayne Rust (2000), whom I met through Psychotherapists and Counsellors for Social Responsibility, have highlighted adults' resistance to facing planetary change. Your work on 'Green Care' makes a fundamental link with emotional wellbeing and working with the environment: the subject of another book.

Meanwhile, how schools and multi-disciplinary and multi-agency teams work together to help children's emotional development seems vital, and pressing. . .

Schools cannot avoid 'emotional development'

RH: In many ways schools cannot avoid 'emotional development' – as everybody who attends them is in the thick of it! I am sure that good schools are 'emotionally intelligent' and that they naturally think about these things as part of the day-to-day work. An example from my own family is the way that Personal and Social Education and drama seem to give opportunities that I never had for discussing and exploring things.

In thinking about this chapter, and the role of drama in emotional development, I recently did a ten-minute piece of 'reality research' on my own four children. One was excellent at it and went on to be the lead role in school plays and local theatre productions, and to study film at university; another, who was then doing it in key stage three, thought it was good because 'it's fun', and only disliked it for the homework (to find a definition of "celebration" and print out or draw a picture to show it: 'It's about funerals, birthdays, and stuff like that', I was told). The next I interviewed had mixed views: 'they kind of force you to do stuff you might not want to do', but also said 'it lets you do what you want to do – like a kind of freedom' and considered it a middling kind of lesson. And the other one was not at all keen: 'Absolutely hated it – I'm not that sort of person. Doing all those things in front of people and stuff. Nothing good about it'. Without wanting to make too many revelations about my own children, the one obvious correlation was between how positively they rated it and how extrovert they were. Which might indicate a need to be particularly sensitive to the needs of the introverted children who try to avoid it (who may also be the ones who most 'need' it).

LL: Drama teachers notice some children really baulk at presenting dramatic work to classmates. Holmwood and Stavrou (chapter 3) discuss the differences between drama teaching and dramatherapy. Essentially dramatherapists train to work psychotherapeutically through drama with the client's inner world. An illustration: as onetime Head of Drama in a Tottenham school, I frequently experienced a very unboundaried young man during drama lessons climbing the wall of our school theatre. Drama enables expression and creativity, but for some young people a drama lesson can prove too exposing in front of peers. Dramatherapy, differently, and linked, enables expression within a contained, therapeutic space, with no pressure to have to perform or join in. Trying out and thinking with the therapist and others in the group about different ways of being and behaving, enables empathy and tolerance.

Perhaps you could say a little about aetiology: the kind of reasons why people might become mentally ill. Sometimes there can be a link with difficult, challenging or very withdrawn behaviour in schools.

RH: When human development is disrupted, the psychological, social and economic consequences can reach into every area of an individual's personal and social world, resulting in alienated and chaotic lives and repercussions throughout their communities. The causes of this disruption may cover the whole range of physical, environmental, psychological, social and economic factors: from an unlucky genetic inheritance to a difficult birth, child abuse, inadequate parenting, failed attachment, trauma or emotional deprivation. The causes can also be poverty: material poverty, or the poverty of expectation that leaves individuals feeling powerless to have any impact on the world in which they live.

Some people can emerge from their early experience to live what appear thriving and healthy lives because of educational advantage, or strong constitutions, or having comfortable homes and buoyant families. Overriding differences in class and educational advantage confer some strong constitutions – or a range of poorly understood protective factors – which may be sufficient to enable them to withstand the impact of these environmental failures. However, very many people end up in a situation where they are excluded from mainstream society, rejected by those who might be able to help them, and destined to live lives of unremitting frustration, without the happiness and fulfilment that most of us would consider just – and expect for ourselves and our families.

These individuals, and often their families, have little psychological sense of their place amongst others or where they fit into society. School, working lives and almost any pro-social relationships are difficult or impossible to establish and sustain. They experience the world as a hostile, unhelpful, threatening or undermining environment, living in a marginalized underclass with high levels of substance misuse, self harm, criminality, and suffering severe, enduring and disabling mental distress. People in this situation will often use a considerable range of statutory services to little benefit.

A minority will receive a formal diagnosis of personality disorder and so gain access to appropriate personality disorder intervention services. However, the majority will receive an ambiguous and often prejudicial formulation of their difficulties and will be more likely to meet a range of unsatisfactory public service responses.

LL: Dramatherapists work in schools and hospitals with children whose parents may themselves be diagnosed with mental health issues. Fonagy and Bateman (2006: 18) helpfully discuss difficulties in attachment. Parental ties can be encouraged and supported by dramatherapists and other psychotherapists in schools, as Leigh (chapter 24) describes.

RH: As far as current government policy on personality disorder is concerned, it has sought to achieve three objectives: to improve health and social outcomes, to reduce social exclusion, and to improve public protection. This includes working with: 'emerging personality disorder in children and adolescents'.

LL: The latter sounds particularly important. Irvine Gersch focuses on the importance of listening to children (chapter 22). And providing therapeutic space in schools enables troubled adolescents, even through 'Drop In' breaktimes, to express themselves, to be heard and to feel accepted, more on an even keel.

Manning (2010) comments on the limitations of a diagnosis: how it can in a sense be a power issue (Haigh 2004). Domikles points out (chapter 7) that through a diagnosis funding can then be accessed for dramatherapy. Adolescents like Jake, mentioned in chapter 7, present serious challenges to teachers and sometimes outside school to society. Yet labelling with a diagnosis can be detrimental. There is therefore rather a dilemma. Considerably increased funding for psychotherapists/dramatherapists to work together with teachers and parents in a triangulated approach with schoolchildren would help enormously.

RH: Cross-agency work is a solution. As far as adult mental health is concerned, evidence from the government-funded pilot projects across the country is emerging. Answers do exist, but they do not lie in a traditional mental health treatment model or straightforward social policy. Rather they lie in sophisticated cross-agency work that takes in the experience and expertise from various sectors: including health, social services, offender management, housing, social security and the voluntary sector. Progress also involves new forms of partnership, in personality disorders with service users themselves – where they can feel themselves as active agents in their own recovery, rather than the passive recipient of technical expertise.

This is the very beginning for a field that is more complex than a disease model or unitary interventions can address. At this stage there is a need to continue to encourage evaluated and researched service innovation, and establish a workforce equipped to meet the demand for skilled and specialist intervention. To be effective, this will require closer collaboration across public services to ensure that the relevance of personality disorders (whether or not that actual term is used) is understood and informs policy, strategy and service provision. This can be better achieved by education working closely with the fields of health, social care and criminal justice.

Children's emotional development

RH: After birth, what happens to every child is emotional development. The lucky ones, given 'good enough' parenting, will emerge sufficiently well-adjusted to enjoy a 'normal' life. The constitutionally disadvantaged ones may survive without long- lasting consequences if they have extra input for their emotional development – perhaps including professional help.

Any child who has a bad experience of emotional development, without sufficient internal or environmental protection against it, will end up at risk of having an unhelpful view of themselves, other people, and the world: possibly leading to a personality disorder. Some with a fortunate or strong constitution may be protected, and able to later cope as adults, because they have had some reasonably nurturant relationships with which to develop a less distorted view of themselves, others and the world. Those who start life with a congenital disadvantage are very much likelier to suffer a severe impact from an inadequate emotional environment.

LL: Family life is linked intrinsically from when children are small. Schools can help children learn: that is their work. What seems to help, I'd suggest, is where psychotherapists and arts therapists can enable good boundaries for children's sense of self. I have seen that boundaries seem to hold a key to enabling more useful, clearer relationships.

RH: Interesting. Environmental conditions (including how much a child feels loved) also change over time. Also, the way a child behaves, perhaps because of the brain it has inherited, will have an effect on, for example, whether it is punished or comforted. To add complexity, we can include the effect of human agency at every point: conscious or unconscious choices that may be adaptive or maladaptive are made at every decision point in a parent's and a child's life. These will have an impact on thoughts, feelings, behaviour and subsequent choices – in an unpredictable way with multiple dependent and independent variables. This is closer to chaos theory than a deterministic model.

'The Quintessence' developmental model

A developmental model that describes the necessary experience for 'fairly normal' emotional development can be constructed. This we can call 'primary emotional development': primary because it is the first time it happens to people, because it is in childhood, and because it is a collection of fundamental human psychological processes.

The five-experience model ('The Quintessence', Haigh 1999) works in a suitably flexible and adaptable way, which puts several psychological theories together into these sequential and overlapping experiences:

- attachment (feeling connected, and belonging)
- containment (feeling safe)
- communication (feeling heard, in a culture of openness)
- inclusion (feeling involved, as part of the whole)
- agency (feeling empowered with a solid sense of self).

LL: Your model fits well with this book's title, which suggests we are on the same walk along challenging terrain, with a rather good view ahead. Dramatherapy works to enable children and parents to feel a sense of attachment, of creativity, and to become more aware of their feelings – a sense of self: this book shows that. Dramatherapy groups certainly help adolescents' sense of inclusion and agency.

RH: If this defines primary emotional development, secondary emotional development is what we can engineer to happen if it went wrong 'first time round'. It is the intention of the therapeutic environment to recreate these five conditions.

LL: As you said earlier, how much better if the emphasis is on children's development rather than on later developmental difficulties.

RH: Some schools can be demotivating. This can be as much true of a school (where children feel demotivated and uninspired), an office (where there is a continual feeling of suspicion and fear), a company (where workers constantly feel there is an 'us and them' relationship with the bosses) as of a family or therapeutic community: any setting where a group of people are emotionally engaged in some sort of developmental task together. This implies that these concepts of secondary emotional development are not only about specialist hospital or prison units for treating personality disorders – they are about everyday life, and struggling to try and meet needs that we all have as we go about our normal lives.

LL: We both agree that among the struggles of everyday life, which we all go through, dramatherapy with play therapy and the creative arts therapies have something special to offer children in schools.

RH: Yes, the creative therapies and arts therapies such as dramatherapy, can 'reach the parts that other therapies cannot reach'.

When considerable preventive work, or therapeutic work while children are still at the age where the primary emotional development is taking place . . . the personality is not yet 'set' – and perhaps abuses, traumas and deprivations can be put right before they colour somebody's emergence into adulthood.

And for this, the creative and expressive therapies have a particularly important role to play. The first two positive 'emotional experiences' – attachment and containment – are the overwhelmingly predominant ones in somebody's early life – before words mean anything, and when all experience is focused on infantile and pre-verbal life. In their ability to work without needing to formulate experience into words and into 'adult constructions' to make sense of irrational and unconscious thinking, these therapies can 'reach the parts that other therapies cannot reach' and access disturbed areas of experience directly, without the feelings needing to be translated into words and then back into feelings. This is often better done in company of others, so the non-verbal learning is shared, and the whole is well 'contained' through relationships, rather than structures, rules and procedures.

LL: Our case studies and other examples of dramatherapy practice throughout this book, for instance the family work that Mercieca, Dooman and I have detailed, highlight this very phenomenon.

RH: These, of course, are underpinning principles of therapeutic community practice (Kennard 2006 [1998]).

LL: Interesting that we've come full circle back to this parallel of therapeutic communities and schools. Schools can offer the creative arts therapies and play therapy, which enable children's unexpressed and difficult feelings to be expressed, not necessarily through words.

RH: I found something completely different about the way people were with each other in therapeutic communities. I learnt my psychiatry the same as other students who were on traditional wards, but I also got an inkling of something that is very hard to define or put in words. It was something about being allowed to be yourself, about playfulness, and creativity.

LL: That significant parallel again, of playfulness and creativity . . . It is not the world of cognitive learning, but I think it goes in parallel, in tandem with it.

RH: Thirty years after qualifying, I am the consultant psychiatrist in a therapeutic community, and have been for 20 years. Throughout my working life I have always been wondering just what 'it', this intangible quality, is.

LL: Thank you Rex. Your contribution enables readers to think from a valuable sociological and psychological overall perspective about the spectrum of mental health and about the importance of good-enough emotional wellbeing for children and young people in schools.

RH: The spectrum of mental health is 'a spectrum upon which we all sit somewhere'.

Now we only need to get rid of the ghastly 'personality disorder' term itself, and make the opinion-makers and media understand that it is a spectrum upon which we all sit somewhere: 'everybody has a personality, and nobody is perfect'.

Bibliography

Department of Health (2005) *Mental Health of Children and Young People in Great Britain, 2004*. Available at: http://www.dh.gov.uk/en/Publicationsandstatistics/Publications/PublicationsStatistics/DH_4118332 (Accessed 25 September 2011).

Fonagy P. and Bateman, A. (2006) *Mentalisation-Based Treatment for Borderline Personality Disorder: A Practical Guide*. Oxford: Oxford University Press.

Foulkes, E. F. (1990) *Selected Papers of S. H. Foulkes: Psychoanalysis and Group Analysis*. London: Karnac.

Haigh, R. (1999) 'The quintessence of a therapeutic environment', in Penelope Campling and Rex Haigh (eds.), *Therapeutic Communities: Past, Present and Future*. London: Jessica Kingsley, 246–257.

Haigh, R. (2004) 'The problem with Personality Disorder'. Address to Reading Therapies Group.

Kennard, D. (2006 [1998]) *An Introduction to Therapeutic Communities. Community, Culture and Change 1*. London: Jessica Kingsley.

Laing, D. (1990 [1959]) *The Divided Self: An Existential Study of Sanity and Madness*. London: Penguin.

Manning, N. (2010) 'Therapeutic communities: a problem or a solution for psychiatry? A sociological view'. *British Journal of Psychotherapy* 26 (4), 434–443.

Prentice, H. (2003) 'Cosmic walk: Awakening the ecological self'. *Psychotherapy and Politics International* 1 (1), 32–46.

Rust, M. J. (2000) Psychotherapy on the Titanic: PCSR conference June 2000. London. Available at: http://www.rainforestinfo.org.au/deep-eco/web/Web6/titanic.htm (Accessed 30 January 2011).

Conclusions

Irvine Gersch

In this book we have aimed to explain something about dramatherapy and its use with children and young people, in schools and educational settings. Examples of the use of dramatherapy have been provided in individual chapters, which illustrate these very possibilities.

The book has been divided into five main parts:

I Introduction
II Case studies
III Collaborative partners in schools and beyond
IV Evidence and outcomes
V Future possibilities

This reflects the thinking of the editors about 'the case for dramatherapy'. Having set out the educational and national scene, in part I, the book goes on, in part II, to provide a range of vivid and colourful examples demonstrating the fascinating and creative ways in which dramatherapy is practised by highly experienced and renowned practitioners.

Part III has focused, importantly, on collaborative partners in schools and beyond, since it is the view of the editors that, for dramatherapy to be effective in today's world of multi-agency working, such partnerships are critical.

One of the first questions raised by those non-practitioners interested in finding out more about dramatherapy or, indeed, before agreeing to provide it in schools and educational settings is 'Does it work?' Allied to this, questions about the ethical context and health and safety issues are typically posed. Therefore, part IV of this book is devoted to a discussion of the evidence and outcomes of dramatherapy, which is a growing area of research. Ethical issues are reviewed in chapter 1 and the reader is directed to the link to the BADth website, which contains a detailed Code of Conduct, and to that of the Health Professional Council (HPC), membership of which is mandatory for dramatherapists.

The essential case made in this book, at its heart, is that dramatherapy is an under-used source of help and support for children. This under-use of dramatherapy in our schools is notable and disappointing, particularly when there is growing evidence of its value and benefit. Perhaps there has been some confusion about the difference between drama teaching and dramatherapy, although it is possible to speculate other factors that might explain why dramatherapy is not more widely and universally commissioned in our schools. In any event, the reasons for this merit serious further study.

Notwithstanding, I feel strongly that the lack of dramatherapy provision is regrettable, and that its under-use, coupled with somewhat limited awareness about the nature and benefits of this therapy, is a loss to children and young people, a loss to families and a loss to schools and educational agencies.

However, the world is changing. Schools are about to gain greater freedom of choice. At the time of writing, we are anticipating a Green Paper that will review special educational needs, and there is a much greater acceptance of different types of therapy and the positive emotional welfare of children. In addition, the government is planning a major organisational review of the NHS, commencing in 2011. The upsurge of interest in schools wishing to develop wellbeing curricula, the recognition of the importance of happiness and personal learning, creativity, communication, emotional literacy and wellbeing are all indicators of this change. Indeed, this is reflected in the full title of this book, which is *Dramatherapy with Children, Young People and Schools: Enabling creativity, sociability, communication and learning.*

I hope that this changing scene will enable new and positive links between those offering to provide dramatherapy and those wishing to arrange and commission this in schools, thereby extending opportunities for children and young people.

This book has aspired to raise awareness about the case for dramatherapy, through telling its story in some detail, in the hope that this awareness will lead to some action on the part of those who can make a difference; this may be policy makers, managers and those involved in CAMHS and social care, headteachers, school staff, school governors.

The book has also been written as a resource for aspiring dramatherapists, students of dramatherapy and the other arts therapies, including art and music therapy, dance and movement therapy, play therapy and psychotherapy. Indeed, the book would be of value to any professional working within the health, social care and education system, including teachers, teaching assistants, psychologists and those who work in CAMHS, school nurses, social workers, and all those professions who work with children and young people. We hope too that it will be of interest to parents, young people and anyone who wishes to learn more about this creative and exciting profession.

Some useful addresses and websites

Compiled by Deborah Haythorne

The British Association of Dramatherapists
Featuring the Code of Practice and links to Education Committee
The British Association of Dramatherapists
Waverley
Battledown Approach
Cheltenham
Gloucestershire
GL52 6RE
Telephone: +44 (0)1242 235 515
Email: enquiries@badth.org.uk
Website: http://www.badth.org.uk

Sesame Institute (UK and International)
Sesame Institute (UK & International)
27 Blackfriars Road
London
SE1 8NY
Telephone: +44 (0)20 7633 9690
Email: info@sesame-institute.org
Website: http://www.sesame-institute.org

Health Professions Council
Health Professions Council
Park House
184 Kennington Park Road
London
SE11 4BU
Website: http://www.hpc-uk.org

Roundabout
Roundabout
Cornerstone House
14 Willis Road

Croydon
CR0 2XX
Telephone: +44 (0)20 8665 0038
Email: roundabout@cornerstonehouse.org.uk
Website: http://www.roundaboutdramatherapy.org.uk

Playing Matters
59 Defoe House
Barbican
London
EC2Y 8DN
Telephone: +44 (0)20 7628 1763
Email: brenda@playingmatters.co.uk
Website: http://www.playingmatters.co.uk

TRAINING COURSES

Sesame
MA Drama and Movement Therapy
Sesame
The Central School of Speech and Drama
Embassy Theatre
Eton Avenue
London
NW3 3HY
Telephone: +44 (0)20 7722 8183
Contact person: Richard Hougham
Email: r.hougham@cssd.ac.uk
Website: http://www.cssd.ac.uk/shadow/content/ma-drama-and-movement-therapy-sesame?story=0

Roehampton University
MA Dramatherapy
MA (Upgrade) Dramatherapy
Roehampton University
80 Roehampton Lane
London
SW15 5SL
Telephone: +44 (0)20 8392 3807
Contact person: Henru Seebohm
Email: H.Seebohm@Roehampton.ac.uk
Website: http://www.roehampton.ac.uk/postgraduate-courses/dramatherapy

University of Derby
MA in Dramatherapy
Department of Therapeutic Arts and Complementary Medicines
University of Derby Western Road
Mickleover
Derby
DE3 9GX
Telephone: +44 (0)1332 594056
Contact person: Drew Bird
Email: d.p.bird@derby.ac.uk
Website: http://www.derby.ac.uk/dramatherapy-ma

Anglia Ruskin University
MA Dramatherapy
Anglia Ruskin University
Music and Performing Arts Department
East Road
Cambridge CB1 1PT
Telephone: +44 (0)845 271 3333
Admissions: hannah.thurston@anglia.ac.uk
Academic enquiries: ditty.dokter@anglia.ac.uk
Website: http://www.anglia.ac.uk/ruskin/en/home/faculties/alss/deps/mpa.html

Index